MW00990446

Dear Larissa

613.907
AKA
(par)

Sexuality Education for Girls Ages 11-17

Cynthia G. Akagi

GYLANTIC PUBLISHING COMPANY

Littleton, Colorado

JAN 1995

Penn Hills Library
240 Aster Street
Pittsburgh, PA 15235-2099

Although the author has done research to ensure the accuracy and completeness of the information and drawings contained in this book, the author and publisher assume no responsibility for errors, inaccuracies, omissions, or any other inconsistency herein. Data contained herein are the most complete and accurate available as this book goes to press. Please bear in mind that meanings can vary due to personal interpretation.

To order additional copies:
GYLANTIC PUBLISHING COMPANY
P.O. Box 2792
Littleton, Colorado 80161-2792
1-800-828-0113
Add $2.00 to each order for shipping and handling

Printed in the United States by Gilliland Printing, Inc.
The text is printed with soy ink.

Copyright © 1994 by Cynthia G. Akagi

Trademarks
Depo-Provera® is the trademark of The Upjohn Co., Kalamzoo, MI
Norplant System® is the trademark of Wyeth-Ayerst, Philadelphia, PA

All rights reserved. No part of this publication may be reproduced or transmitted in any form or by an means, electronic or mechanical, photocopy, recording or any information storage or retrieval system, without permission in writing from the publisher.

Library of Congress Cataloging-in-Publication-Data

Akagi, Cynthia G., 1959-
    Dear Larissa : sexuality education for girls ages 11-17 / Cynthia G. Akagi.
        p. cm.
    Includes bibliographical references and index.
    ISBN 1-880197-10-3 : $12.95
    1. Sex instruction for girls. 2. Sex instruction for teenagers.
[1. Sex instruction for girls.]   I. Title.
HQ51.A34   1994
613.9'07—dc20   93-44518
                                                            CIP
                                                            AC

Dedication

To my sisters, Chris and Carla,
in memory of boys, dating, sex and love.

Acknowledgments

To the following people I extend many thanks. This book would not have been completed without their support: my husband, Mark; editors, Cheryl Metzger, Jane Moore, and Marcia Malott; illustrators, Angie Di Cicco and Wanda Heberling; Juanita L. Smith, Director, Shawnee County Teen Pregnancy Prevention Program, Topeka, Kansas; Dr. M. Betsy Bergen, sexuality professor, Kansas State University, Manhattan, KS; Larry Siegel, sexuality educator, Del Ray Beach, FL; Jill Bradney, sexuality educator, and her students, Perry-Lecompton High School, Perry, KS; Vicki Manns, sexuality educator and her students, French Middle School, Topeka, KS; Joyce Volmut, former director, Shawnee County Family Planning Clinic, Topeka, KS; the mother/daughter critique teams which space doesn't allow me to list individually; my Wednesday night writing colleagues; the many friends who shared their teen memories with me; God for the gift of writing.

Table of Contents

FOREWORD TO PARENTS

Do you find it difficult to talk to your daughter about growing up and dating? Do you feel embarrassment about discussing sex and fear your own inadequacy about sexual
knowledge? Are you concerned about your daughter having
sexual relationships and becoming a pregnant teenager?

Are your wishes for her to grow up with a healthy body and
mind, to get the best out of life in terms of lasting friendships
and loving relationships, and to positively accept and respect
her sexuality as a basic part of her personality? Do you wish
her to develop the values and attitudes that will help her become a successful, healthy and happy adult, perhaps someday
choosing a mate wisely and experiencing motherhood with
her own daughter?

If these questions are reflective of your thoughts and concerns, how can you communicate them to your daughter?

For most parents one thing is certain: talking with your kids
about your values and attitudes concerning growing up, dating, relationships and sex is never easy. Yet, parents are the
first and foremost sexuality educators of their daughters,
whether they teach poorly or well, or even if the topic is
never mentioned aloud.

Dear Larissa by Cynthia G. Akagi is a book for you to read
and then give to your daughter to be read and, hopefully, discussed with you throughout her teen years.

Lovingly written by a mother to her daughter, *Dear Larissa* is a compilation of letters about growing up—body changes, boys, dating, love and sex—that provide accurate, positive information spelled out in useful detail in a comfortable, conversational style.

The letters are neither preachy, put-downs nor boring versions of "when I was your age." Rather they are written as if you were talking to your daughter. The mother really talks with Larissa as she shares some of her own growing-up experiences and her sexual and personal values, together with accurate, pertinent sexuality information.

That sexual feelings are natural and healthy is the theme of the book and the author is commended for her successful integration of that theme within a teen girl-boy perspective. She believes that children taught to value their sexuality, and given correct information about body maturation, conception, pregnancy and development of dating and love relationships will make responsible, mature choices about their sexual activity throughout their teen years.

The mother's letters to Larissa do not advocate teen sexual intercourse; neither do they say "just say no." The message is: sex changes dating and the rules of dating, impressing upon Larissa that her decisions about sexual activity should not be made lightly. Letter 20 provides detailed information about the advantages and disadvantages of birth control methods and where to purchase commercial ones. The letter emphasizes that when having intercourse to use birth control every time.

Dear Larissa closes with these final thoughts: be your own person, love yourself for who you are, keep your dreams, cherish your sexuality, care for your body and enjoy your teen years. "I will always love you and I'm proud to be your mom."

Dr. M. Betsy Bergen
Kansas State University

Foreword To Daughters

Dear Larissa is a book for you to read and hopefully discuss with your mom. Moms often find it difficult to talk with their daughters. Your mom may find it difficult to talk with you, especially now that you are growing up. You can help her overcome this difficulty.

Your mom may have given this book to you. It is a group of twenty-four letters about growing up—body changes, boys, dating, love and sex—written by a mother to her daughter. *Dear Larissa* provides positive useful information about lots of questions you have and will continue to have throughout your teenage years.

The letters are neither preachy, put-downs nor boring versions of "when I was your age," but rather they are written as if your mother were talking to you. There is solid information about boys and why they act the way they do, about dating relationships with boys, about love and sex and the decisions you will need to make.

You can learn about other topics, too, whenever you have a need for the information. How to care and protect yourself from sexual abuse and sexually transmitted diseases is included as well as birth control methods and where to get them.

Dear Larissa closes with some final thoughts that every mother has for her daughter and that your mother has for you.

Dr. M. Betsy Bergen
Kansas State University

Author's Note

When researching this book, the number one comment I heard from daughters regarding their mothers was: "I need my mother to have faith in me. My asking a sex question doesn't mean I'm going to do what I asked about. I simply want a correct answer, so I know if what I'm hearing at school is the truth or a lie."

On the flip side, mothers said: "It's difficult accepting the reality that my little girl is becoming a sexual person. I want her to have good dating experiences. I don't want to see her get hurt."

The birth control and teen pregnancy information in this book has been explained in a context suitable for pre-teens.

Some parents may think: "I can't let my eleven-or-twelve-year-old read about teen pregnancy and birth control." If you want to impress upon your children the seriousness of teen pregnancy, that message should begin at the preteen age level. If you wait until your daughter is sixteen to talk to her, she will have already formed her beliefs regarding dating behavior.

Some aspects of dating have changed since I was a teen, while others have remained the same. Throughout the book I have included quotes from teens today regarding their feelings about dating, sex and love.

I hope this book will be a good beginning for both of you.

Letter 1

Dear Larissa,

Dear Larissa,

Your preteen and teen years can be some of the best times of your life—school, girlfriends, boys. . . .

But they can also be trying times. Your body will be developing into an adult body. You'll be shaping who you are as a person. You'll be learning about relationships, dating, sex and love.

I think about you growing up. That's why I'm giving you these letters. I was once a teenager and I experienced some of the same things you'll go through—including relationships and dating.

I could never give you all the sexuality information you need in one sitting, nor could you remember it all. The best way to give you sexuality information is to write it down. You can read these letters in private and have time to think about the information. Maturing into adulthood is about taking responsibility for your body and forming a set of personal values about your sexuality.

As a parent, it's my responsibility to prepare you for your new sexuality and your changing body. The truth is you're not a little girl anymore. Your body is already beginning to mature; you're developing breasts, body hair, and having periods.*

Time will pass quickly. There's junior high, then high school, graduation, and moving out on your own. . .on-the-job training, a trade school or college, a job, a career, and/or marriage. And through it all, there will be boys, guys and men.

You may fall for someone your freshman year only to find out he isn't all that great once you get to know him. You may begin dating someone your senior year and realize you'd like to spend the rest of your lives together. Or, you may be so focused on school and getting ready for life beyond graduation that you don't "seriously" fall for a guy until after high school or college.

We are all different. Each one of us matures at a different rate. Look at the girls in your class. Some girls are extremely interested in boys; other girls like boys, but they also have other interests. What do you think of guys right now?

In terms of body changes and teen sex and love, you will learn more in your teens than at any other time in your life.

---

* Some of you reading this haven't yet started your period. Most girls start between eleven and seventeen years of age. Whatever age you start your period will be normal for you. Everyone's body has its own time-table of development.

That's why it's important for you to have the facts about growing up. With correct information, you can make responsible decisions about love and sex. Without good decision-making you can fall into harmful situations—like catching a sexually transmitted disease (STD) or having an unwanted pregnancy. Having the facts will enable you to enjoy your teen years and have control over your body.

Larissa, I don't intend for these letters to replace our talking to each other. In fact, these letters should help us both feel more comfortable talking about sex and love, and they will also be good reference material for you throughout high school.

Please know that you can come to me with any question or problem—even if it's embarrassing to you. Teens should be able to ask their parents questions. If I don't know the answer, I'll help you find the answer.

Some of the information in these letters you won't need until you're older. You can refer back to that information when you need it. But because of the peer pressure teens face today, I want to give you all the facts now.

Here's to you and your teen years—school, friends, life!

I love you,
Mom

_____

_____

_____

_____

_____

_____

LETTER 2

A HISTORY OF SEX SINCE GRANdMA WAS A TEEN

Dear Larissa,

Before I discuss body changes, boys, and dating, I want to give you some background on the history of sex education in our family and in America. This should help you understand why it's important that you and I talk about sexuality issues.

One day—I was either twelve or thirteen—I asked your grandmother about sex. Now this question hit your grandmother like a brick wall falling on her. Grandma was not prepared to talk to me about sex because her mother had not talked to her about sex, nor had her mother before that.

Before the 1980s, sex was not discussed in most American homes. It was also not taught in school—except for the "menstruation film" for girls and perhaps a quick anatomy lesson given to the boys in gym class. Our society was uncomfortable talking about sex. Teens were regarded as children—not developing, sexual persons. Though teens had normal sexual feelings, they were told those feelings were wrong or dirty. Few teens were told that maturing into their adult bodies was a normal, healthy growth process.

In the fifties and early sixties many girls and a good number of guys did not have intercourse until they married. Girls were afraid of becoming pregnant—and for good reason. There was no effective means of birth control for women. Unwed mothers were outcasts and abortions were illegal and dangerous.

In 1960 a group of doctors created "the Pill"—the oral contraceptive. The creation of oral contraceptives was a historical step in both women's rights and reproductive choice. With oral contraceptives women could now effectively space their children so they could be better mothers; or postpone child-rearing until they completed college or vocational school.

Unfortunately, the changing sixties introduced the idea of casual sex to society—if you liked someone, have sex with them. Your Grandma, frightened of the new sexual attitudes, shut up and wouldn't talk to me about sex at all. This only left me with more questions and more confused.

If only Grandma had felt comfortable enough to sit down and explain to me that, yes, some people have sex before they are married, but there are serious pregnancy and STD risks of casual sex (as the sixties and seventies' children soon found out). There were also emotional and self-respect issues—like a person using another person for sex and then dumping the person—and that still happens a lot.

But with little sexuality information being taught in the home or at school, most of my friends and I learned about sex by experimenting. Experimenting is the wrong way to learn. The lessons are filled with incorrect information and serious mistakes. Several girls became pregnant. Some had abortions. Others carried their pregnancies to term and gave their babies up for adoption. Adoption was utilized much more in the seventies than it is today.

Larissa, your world today is different. Your world is exciting because society is realizing that teens are maturing young people who need to know about body changes, love, sex, and relationships.

Today, STDs affect one out of every three teens, in both country and city schools.

Your world is also terrifying. One wrong choice and you can become pregnant or contract a STD or AIDS. That's why it's vital that you have the sexuality information you need to make responsible decisions for yourself when you begin dating.

Happily, I can give you this book and you can come to me with any type of question and I'll answer it for you—Grandma would be proud of us.

Love and hugs,
Mom

L ETTER 3

Your Changing Body and Changing Feelings

Dear Larissa,

It is quite miraculous the way our bodies change from child bodies to adult bodies. We females develop breasts, our hips widen, we grow body hair, and start our periods. Guys also change. They grow body hair, their chests, testes, and penises develop, their voices change and they begin shaving. These physical changes are called "puberty." Puberty normally takes place between ten and sixteen years of age, but each person begins puberty according to her or his body's own time table.

Your new body is more complex than your old body. To become comfortable with your new body and keep yourself healthy, you need to become familiar with your sexual anatomy. Because more and more schools are teaching reproduction in health class, you may already know some of this

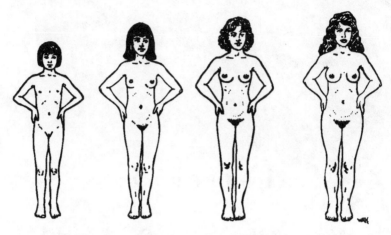

Female Development From Girl To Woman

information. But by having all the information here in these letters, you can refer to it when you have questions.

Hormones—chemical messengers from your brain—begin the change toward adulthood. They signal your body to start equipping you with the physical capability to one day have children. The word puberty means capable of reproduction. During puberty your body is maturing from your reproductively immature, child body into your adult, sexual body. These changes can be exciting and embarrassing all at the same time.

When your body begins changing, you may feel excited, uncomfortable, or self-conscious. Changes are happening to your body and you have no control over them. Body hair appears, your breasts grow, you get your period. Help! Help! Larissa you're not alone. Everyone feels a little weird and self-conscious when their bodies begin developing, including your Dad and I when we were teens.

I was in the sixth grade when I discovered I was developing breasts and growing pubic hair. At first I didn't tell anyone. It was my secret. Did you feel different when you discovered your body was changing?

If you're ever sitting in class worrying about yourself, look around the room. Everyone will go through the same body changes you're going through. Some of your classmates may not be showing changes yet, but you can be sure their growth hormones are readying for attack.

Maturing into your sexual adult body is a natural, healthy process. There is nothing dirty or bad about your body changing. During puberty your body's sexual hormones awaken so that you can:

* enjoy and nurture a mature relationship through physical touch and

* have children when you are an adult .

To understand your new body, you need to take a good look at yourself. You may want to touch your body parts and study yourself in a mirror. Boys grow up holding their

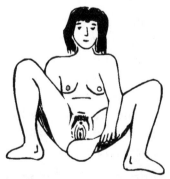

Girl Examining Vulva With Hand Mirror

penises to urinate, so they're usually more at ease touching their bodies than we females. We also need to know where our body parts are and what they feel like. Being familiar with your body will enable you to take care of your body, and there is nothing embarrassing about taking care of yourself.

After you read this letter, if you want to talk about a particular body change, or you have questions about body growth, ask me. If I don't know the answers to your questions, I'll help you find the answers.

Preteen girls are most concerned with breast and body hair development and starting their periods. Later on, it's sexual feelings that concern girls. We'll discuss those too, but first things first. . . . Whatever feelings you first have—happy, scared, anxious, self-conscious—any of those feelings are okay. Everyone who has experienced puberty has had all or some of those feelings at one time. How do you feel right now? How do your girlfriends feel about their changing bodies?

With an adult body come adult responsibilities—birth control and STD protection.

While your body is maturing, Larissa, your emotions and thought processes are also maturing. You want to be part of the crowd, yet you want to be your own person. You want responsibility, but you don't want responsibility. You feel one way about a person or issue today, and tomorrow you totally change your mind. You want to do things by yourself and on your own, but you also want me around if you need help, or if life becomes difficult.

This emotional maturing is called "adolescence"—your mental maturing into adulthood. Adolescence lasts for several years, normally from age eleven through your early twenties. Adolescence is a critical growth process. It's the process by which you shape your adult personality and values—how you'll interact with others as an adult.

Unfortunately during adolescence your hormones, working on your body development, also affect your emotions. That's why teens can be moody—slight mood changes as well as serious mood swings. Knowing that hormones are causing your mood swings can help you cope with your feelings. And it's always good to talk about your feelings. You can keep a journal, talk with a close friend, and I'm here if you want to talk to me.

If you feel extremely blah, tired, sad or brooding—you should talk with a school counselor, therapist, or doctor. A physical or emotional problem may be causing your depression. Feeling depressed is no fun. Your mental health is equally important as your physical health and one can affect the other.

In addition to physical and emotional growth, you will also experience new sexual feelings —a sexual adolescence.

In stage one (grade school) you begin discovering the sexual world around you. You may like dirty jokes and become curious about the sex and love you see on TV and in the movies. In grade school I remember leafing through clothing catalogs looking at the men's and women's underwear sections.

In the second stage of sexual awakening (junior high/middle school), your interest in boys will probably increase. You may like romance stories. You may dream of your favorite movie star, singer, or a certain guy in school. When I was in the seventh grade, I got my period, my first real boyfriend, and my first real kiss. Of course in the eighth grade my boyfriend and I broke up—but that's another story. In junior high some guys want to date but others are shy or unsure about dating.

During the first and second stages of sexual adolescence children and preteens may play "Doctor" with the same sex (two girls together, two boys together). These games are a normal expression of sexual curiosity; you are curious about your body. Playing them as a child or preteen does not mean you are a homosexual or an over-sexed person.

The final stage of adolescent sexual awareness comes in high school. Your body is almost fully developed. Your sexual feelings are more intense. You may think about sex often, then wonder if you think about it too much. But nothing is wrong.

The following are sexuality questions we each try to answer at different times during our lives.

- What is my sexual identity? Am I tough, feminine, or a mixture of both?

- Am I okay looking? Am I sexy?

- Do I think about sex a lot? Do I not care about sex much right now? (Both feelings are normal.)

- What are my sexual beliefs and values? What do I think about people making out? What do I think about intercourse?

- Am I heterosexual (attracted to males) or homosexual (attracted to my own female sex)?

The majority of girls and guys in your school will be heterosexual—attracted to the other sex. But some people are homosexual—they are attracted to people of their own sex. Homosexual men are called gays. Homosexual women are called lesbians, though the word "gay" is used to describe both homosexual men and women. You can't tell if someone is gay merely by their looks or how they act. Guys who have feminine characteristics and girls with masculine characteristics are not necessarily homosexuals. In fact, some male sports heroes and some female fashion models may be homosexual. Some researchers believe that people are born with a genetic trait for homosexuality. Other researchers believe that family and social environment influence sexual orientation.

Except for their sexual preference, homosexuals are ordinary people like you and me. Gays have families, friends, talents, dreams, goals, successes, and disappointments. They work in sports, government, industry, religion, the arts, teaching, and the medical community. However, some people don't accept gays and lesbians as equal human beings.

School is especially tough on teens who think they may be homosexual. They wonder if they should act "straight" (heterosexual) because everyone else is into girl-guy dating. They often feel alone, isolated and confused. Many homosexual teens don't feel safe talking to their friends or their parents for fear they will be shunned, teased, and rejected.

But homosexual teens shouldn't be shunned. If you suspect someone in your circle of friends may be homosexual you could be a friend he or she can talk with. If you are uncomfortable being around homosexual people, you don't have to be best friends with them. Be respectful in the same way you desire respect from your peers for your sexual values. You can read more about homosexuality from books available at the public library or local bookstores.

No person, regardless of color or sex preference, should be discriminated against or shunned. We're all equal human beings. You or I could have easily been born homosexual rather than heterosexual—or born to a family with a different skin color or culture. Our differences are what makes each of us unique and interesting. What do you think of people who are different from you? I'm usually curious about how they live, what they think, and what their values are.

Larissa, your sexual values emerge from your sexuality—how you feel about yourself and your body. Your sexuality is directly tied to your self-esteem—how you feel about your whole self. Your self-esteem determines your outlook on life and how you get along in the world—the relationships you have with family, friends, and co-workers.

We'll talk more about self-esteem and relationships in my letters on dating. Now, you need to become comfortable with your sexuality by studying your body and learning how your reproductive and sexual anatomy works.

You should feel comfortable with your sexuality, Larissa. The only time sex isn't healthy is:

- when a person uses sex to hurt, abuse, or dominate another person,

- when you have intercourse before you're emotionally able to handle the intimacy or use birth control and STDs protection to protect yourself against unplanned pregnancies, STDs, and AIDS,

- when having sex is against your religious or moral values,

- when you become so obsessed with sex that it dominates your life.

Though there may be certain times in your teens when you think you are obsessed with sex, it usually only seems that way and doesn't require a counselor's attention. But if you become concerned, talk to someone.

At first you may feel modest and self-conscious about your new body. That's normal, and modesty is appropriate in public places and social settings. Most of us feel more comfortable walking down a crowded street with our clothes on rather than off.

Mom, you say I should feel good about my body, but I can count at least three things that really bug me. I wish I had longer legs, blond hair instead of brown hair, and a smaller nose.

Larissa, all of us have things we'd like to change about our appearance, and we often compare ourselves with other people. I have always wanted to be twenty pounds thinner and have hair like my friend Ginny. But I don't have hair like hers, nor will my body ever be twenty pounds thinner.

Your body is only a covering for the you inside. We just waste time when we compare our bodies to other's. Your smile and personality will make you more successful and win you more friends than any fashion magazine body in the world.

My next few letters illustrate body development and give you information on how to take care of your body. I included breast development, menstruation (periods), concep-

tion and pregnancy and other information about your
body. Keep reading.

Take care,
Mom

_____

_____

_____

_____

_____

_____

_____

_____

LETTER 4

Body Talk—BREASTS

Dear Larissa,

There are many slang names for breasts—boobs, titties, hooters, knockers. Our breasts have caused us all concern at one time or another.

"Will my breasts ever grow?" "Mine are growing too much." "My breasts are too small." "My breasts are too large." "When can I wear a bra?" "Do I have to wear a bra?" "If I don't wear a bra will my breasts sag?" "What if I don't like getting breasts?" "Why do guys tease us about our breasts and talk about them behind our backs?" Adults make comments too, without thinking how those comments feel to us. The reason guys tease is that guys like breasts—and I'll tell you more about that later.

At first you may or may not like the idea of developing breasts. Some girls find it embarrassing; others can't wait. When I started developing in the sixth grade, I liked the idea of having breasts, but I didn't want anyone talking about them or teasing me. Small, medium or large, whether you like them at first or not, breasts are part of your sexual anatomy.

As a child your breasts are flat except for your nipple and areola. The nipple is the small, raised portion in the center of your breast and the areola is the ring of skin around the nipple (see illustration on page 22). When females begin to mature, they experience five stages of breast development. Every girl develops at a time that is right for her body. You may begin developing as early as age ten or as late as age sixteen.

At sometime during breast development, you may experience tender or sore nipples and/or breasts. Though the tenderness can be uncomfortable, it's nothing to worry about and will eventually go away. I don't remember my breasts being tender, but your development may be different.

It's also common in breast development for one breast to grow faster than the other. By stage five, the slower growing breast has usually also matured.

The Mature Breast

At stage five, your breasts will be fully developed, although it's common for women to have one breast that is slightly larger than the other. You may have little hairs around your areolas. If you have them, you can shave them, but they will grow back. Do not pluck them or use chemical removers. Your areola area is sensitive; plucking and chemicals can cause infection.

You may also have inverted nipples and/or nipple fluid. Inverted nipples are puckered in. They sink into the areola instead of sticking out. Many women have inverted nipples.

The Five Stages of Breast Development

Stage 1. Childhood breasts are flat. The only raised part is the nipple.

Stage 2. Breast-bud stage. Milk ducts and fat tissue begin forming under each nipple and areola. The nipples grow larger, the areolas wider, and both become darker in color.

Stage 3. Breasts become more round and full and begin to stand out more. Breasts are often cone-shaped at this stage.

Stage 4. In this stage the areola and nipple form a separate mound that protrudes above the breast. Some girls go through this stage and some don't. If you don't, don't worry.

Stage 5. This is the mature breast. Your breasts are fully developed in accordance with your family heredity. Breasts come in all sizes—round, full, thin, cone-shaped, flat.

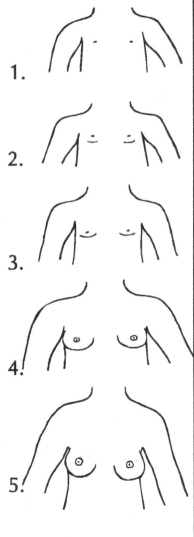

The only time there could be a problem is if an inverted nipple suddenly pulls outward, or vice versa. This doesn't necessarily mean that anything is wrong, but it's a good idea to have it checked by a doctor.

You also may experience a small amount of whitish, clear, slightly yellow, or green fluid draining from the nipple once in a while. This is nipple fluid, and there's nothing to worry about unless it becomes dark brown or has pus in it.

When your breast is fully developed it consists of the outside—nipple and areola, and inside—milk ducts, lobes, alveoli, and fat tissue. This fat tissue is good fat because it protects the inner workings of the breast.

Female breasts serve two purposes.

*   They are sexual parts of the adult body and produce pleasurable feelings when stroked or touched.

*   When we become pregnant, our breasts produce milk for our babies.

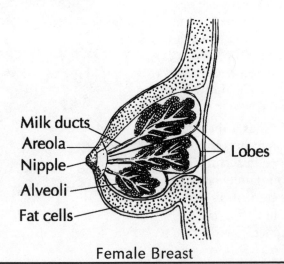

Female Breast

Although you can only see three lobes in the illustration, your breasts are made up of fifteen to twenty-five lobes all packed together in a circle surrounding your areola and nipple. The inside of the breast lobes are tree-like and the alveoli, the tree's leaves, are where milk is made. Breasts only make milk when you have a baby. Milk production does not depend on breast size.

Will your breasts be small, medium, or large? That depends on genetics. The women in our family have medium-size breasts, so that's probably what you'll have. Some girls have small breasts, others large breasts. Despite what advertising would like you to think, large breasts are not better than small breasts. In fact, extremely large-breasted women often have their breasts surgically reduced because the weight of their breasts is tiring, uncomfortable, and causes back problems. I had a large-breasted friend who, at age thirty, had her breasts reduced. She felt so much better afterwards, she wished she had had it done years before.

If you have small breasts, that's great. You may enjoy going braless and you can wear a variety of clothes. If you have medium or large breasts, that's fine too, and there is a different variety of clothing that will look good on you. There is much more to who you are as a person than your breast size.

Bra—To Wear or Not to Wear

Wear a bra or don't wear one? The first time I wore a bra, I felt like I was tied up in a horse bridle. But after I became used to it, I liked it. A bra defined my breasts and made me feel grown-up.

I think you'll find that in school most girls wear bras. Bras define your shape and give your breasts support, much like a jock strap gives a guy's penis support. Some females worry that if they don't wear a bra, their breasts will sag. You shouldn't have to worry about sagging unless you have large breasts or you don't wear a bra for many years.

If and where you wear a bra will be a decision you'll have to make depending on the situation. I feel more comfortable wearing a bra at public gatherings like church, work, and restaurants. I may not wear one around the house. How do you feel about wearing a bra?

When Do You Need a Bra?

When you need a bra is when you think you need one. Some girls like to wear bras even though they're only in stage one of breast development and that's okay. Other girls don't want to wear a bra until they absolutely have to. When the time comes that you think you need a bra, let me know and we'll buy you some.

Bras are available in different sizes and styles. There are one size fits all bras; slightly padded bras if you're just beginning to develop or if you're small breasted and want a fuller look; and extra-support sports bras for athletic activities— dancing, running, horseback riding, volleyball and basketball. What matters is that it supports your breasts and fits comfortably.

Your bra size is determined by your cup size and the number of inches around your chest. Example: 34AAA, 36B, 38D. Cup sizes run from A through D or E, and includes AAA sizes for very small breasts and EE sizes for extra-large breasts. Chest sizes range from twenty-eight inches to forty-four inches. If your chest size is smaller or larger than the twenty-eight to forty-four range, specialty shops carry your size.

Determining Your Correct Bra Size

To determine your bra size, measure yourself with a tape measure as shown below. Write down your measurements, then refer to the chart on the next page for your correct bra size. You can do this by yourself, or I or a girlfriend can help you.

1. Chest size

Measure around your body just under your breasts.

Then add five inches to that measurement.

Example: if you measure twenty-nine inches, add five inches and your chest size is thirty-four inches.

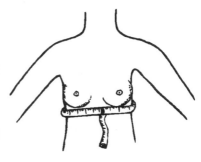

Measuring Chest Size

Figure your chest size here:

_____ inches measured + _5_ inches = _____inches chest size.

2. Cup size

To determine cup size, measure around the widest part of your chest at your nipples and write down your NM (nipple measurement).

Your NM is:

_____inches

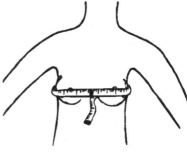

Measuring Cup Size

Now compare your two measurements with the chart on this page to find your bra size. Your bra size is your chest measurement (twenty-eight through forty-four) + your cup size (AAA through EE).

BRA SIZE CHART

CUP   NM (nipple measurement)

AAA—Chest size is larger than nipple measurement (NM).
(Example: Chest 34 is larger than NM size 32 = AAA cup. Bra size: 34 AAA)

AA—Chest size is the same as NM
(Example: Chest 30 and NM 30 = AA cup. Bra size: 30AA)

A—NM is 1 inch larger than chest size.
(Example: NM 31 - chest 30 = 1 inch = A cup. Bra size: 30A)

B—NM is 2 inches larger than chest size.
 (Example: NM 36 - chest 34 = 2 inches = B cup. Bra size: 34B)

C—NM is 3 inches larger than chest size.
 (Example: NM 35 - chest 32 = 3 inches = C cup. Bra size 32C)

D—NM is 4 inches larger than chest size.
(Example: NM 40 - chest 36 = 4 inches = D cup. Bra size is 36D)

E—NM is 5 inches larger than chest size.
 (Example: NM 44 - chest 39 = 5 inches = E cup. Bra size is 39E)

NOTE: *This is approximate cup sizing only. While your breasts are growing you'll want to re-measure yourself each time you buy new bras. You may also want to experiment with different brands and styles of bras to see which style fits you best.*

Boys and Breasts

Breasts are part of our sexual anatomy. Because humans are sexual creatures, guys like girls' breasts in the same way you may think a guy has a nice chest or shoulders. Guys will probably forever whistle at and tease girls. What hurts is when a person, out of cruelty, takes teasing too far. I hope you're never hassled like that, but it could happen.

What can you do? The best thing to do is to ignore the person, and he or she should eventually stop bothering you. Knowing why guys tease girls about their breasts should help you to ignore their remarks and comments. Teasing back usually makes the situation worse.

One other note about breasts: Sexy advertising has placed far too much emphasis on being large breasted. The truth is males appreciate breasts whatever the size. If a guy decides he won't date you or marry you because of your breast size, he isn't worth your time. A person should like you for who you are as a person—not your breast size.

Taking Care of Your Breasts

Taking care of your breasts is relatively easy. Until you begin menstruating, all you need to do is wash your breasts daily with the rest of your body, decide if and when you want to begin wearing a bra, and buy bras that fit comfortably.

After you begin your periods, you should start performing a monthly breast self-exam. What is a breast self-exam? A self-exam is you examining your breasts for any lumps or irregularities that might be signs of cancer or other problems. One of the places females can get cancer is in our breast tissue. The good news is that breast cancer in teens is very rare, and many lumps that women find in their breasts are not cancerous. However, girls who have a history of breast cancer in their families should be especially watchful of breast changes. Also, their doctors may advise beginning regular mammograms earlier than age thirty-five.

If you begin self-exams when you start having periods, it will become a habit, just like brushing your teeth. It will be something you do regularly to keep yourself healthy. Should you ever develop cancer, early detection by monthly self-exams can save your life.

Self-exams only take a few minutes and should be part of your regular routine. They are easy to do after your morning or evening bath or shower. I may be able to get some self-exam cards from our doctor or the health clinic to remind both of us to do our self-exams.

Once you begin menstruating, it's important to do self-breast exams throughout your life. Even Grandma should do monthly exams, as well as have a yearly mammogram. The older a female becomes, the greater her risk of cancer. Opinions differ as to frequency and when to start, but most doctors recommend a yearly mammogram (x-ray of your breasts) after age thirty-five.

The following are breast self-exam instructions. If you like, you can practice the motions while you read this.

Breast Exam—Part 1

Step 1. On the last day of your period stand in front of a mirror with good lighting. The last day of your period is best, as your breasts may be a little lumpy before or during your periods because of slight cyclic duct and tissue swelling. Put your arms at your sides and look at your breasts from the front and side for any unusual moles, sores, de-

pressions, bulges, dark or
red areas or rough-feeling
skin. Check your nipples
and areolas as well. If you
see anything unusual,
check it daily. If it's not
gone in a couple of weeks,
let me know so we can have
a doctor look at it. Put
your hands on your hips
and tighten your upper
chest muscles by pressing
upward and down. Look
for any bulges or dimpling

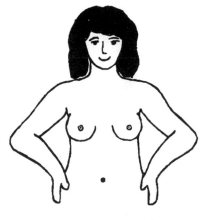

Breast Exam—Step 1

on your breasts. A lump that isn't noticeable otherwise may
show up only with your chest muscles tightened. With
hands still on your hips, turn to each side, looking for the
same thing.

Step 2. Put your hands at
about heart level in front of
your chest. Press your palms
together and look for un-
even muscle contractions,
bulges, or dimpling. Check
the sides of your breasts. If
your breasts are large or
hang down, you'll have to
lift each breast to check its
underside.

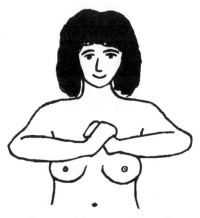

Breast Exam—Step 2

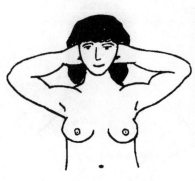

Breast Exam—Step 3

Step 3. Raise your arms, bend your elbows, put your hands behind your head. Again, check the front and both sides for any bulging or dimpling that might indicate a lump. Are you beginning to feel like a body builder striking all these positions in the mirror? Keep going, you're almost finished. When you get the routine down, you'll be able to do a thorough breast self-exam in minutes.

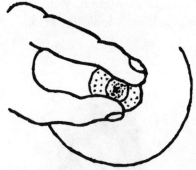

Breast Exam—Step 4

Step 4. Gently squeeze each nipple to see if there is any fluid. Fluid does not necessarily mean there is something wrong, but if there is a lot of it, or it's dark in color or full of pus, tell me. We'll need to have it checked out.

Breast Exam—Part 2

Step 5. Lie down on your bed or your floor. Bend one arm and put it behind your head. This position allows your breasts to spread out, making it easier to check for lumps. Now, using your fingertips, begin in a circular motion and feel each breast. Press down to the chest wall. Feel under

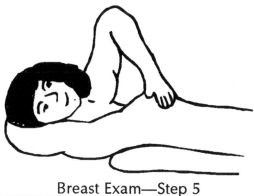

Breast Exam—Step 5

your armpit and your upper chest, too. Then do the same with the other breast. You are feeling for any lump or thickening of the breast. This may sound easy, but most of us have rather bumpy, lumpy breasts anyway and it's easy to mistake ribs, muscles, and ducts for lumps. You may have to use two hands to get an accurate feeling. Using only one hand you may press near a bump and have it slide away. Keep working at it. Once you get an idea of the normal feel of your breasts, any abnormal lumps or bumps should stand out.

If you find anything you think is abnormal, including a nipple suddenly inverting or protruding, let me know. Cancer is rare in young women, but there are non-cancerous conditions that can affect breasts. If the abnormality lasts more than two weeks, we'll need to make a doctor's appointment for you.

Love
Mom

Letter 5

Body Talk—Hair

Dear Larissa,

Both males and females grow body hair. This growth may begin as early as age eight or as late as sixteen. Body hair is part of having an adult body. We females grow hair under our arms and on our legs, on our mons (the mound of skin between our legs), and sometimes around our nipples and above our upper lip. Boys grow hair in these same places and on their face and chest. Body hair helps to protect your body's sensitive areas from dust and dirt particles.

Pubic Hair

Pubic hair grows on the mons—the area of skin just above your genital area. Pubic hair can be any color, blond, brown, black, or red, and not necessarily the same color as your hair color. Some women have a great deal of pubic hair, others don't have much. If the hair on your head turns gray when you age, your pubic hair may also turn gray. The only thing you have to do to care for your pubic hair is to wash your mons daily when you shower or bathe. There are five stages of pubic hair growth for girls. What stage are you in?

Five Stages of Pubic Hair Growth

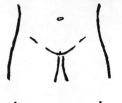

Stage 1
Mons is hairless or there are a few light-colored soft hairs similar to arm hair.

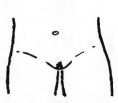

Stage 2
A few darker-colored, some-what curly hairs appear on your mons.

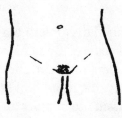

Stage 3
You get more hair and it's thicker, curlier and darker.

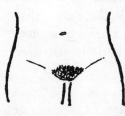

Stage 4
Hair spreads out in a triangular shape, still dark, thick and curly.

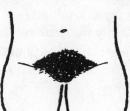

Stage 5
Adult stage. Pubic hair covers a wider area than stage four and is thick and very curly. For some of us, pubic hair grows onto our thighs and/or toward our bellybuttons (navel).

Underarm and Leg Hair

Sometime during puberty you'll also grow underarm hair and more leg hair. In the United States male body hair is considered attractive, while female body hair is usually not considered attractive. For that reason, many women in America routinely remove underarm and leg hair, but generally not pubic hair, except for bikini lines. However, there are some women in America who don't remove their body hair. Removal of your body hair will be up to you. In some countries, women don't shave body hair.

If you decide to shave, at what age should you begin?

Some girls begin before they need to because they want to feel grown-up or fit in with the crowd. However, once you start shaving, your hair will grow back thicker and darker and you'll be removing it for the rest of your life. Girls who mature early may start shaving earlier than their friends. Girls who mature later or have sparse, blond leg hairs, don't have to shave until they're older. If you decide to remove your leg and underarm hair you won't need to begin until it really bothers you.

Removing Underarm and Leg Hair

Shaving

Shaving is inexpensive and the least allergic way to remove body hair. When shaving you can use a disposable or electric razor. Make sure the blades are smooth, sharp and free from nicks, rust or soap build-up.

When using disposable razors, lightly lather your legs and underarms with shaving cream or soap before you shave. Shave slowly and smoothly. When you hurry, it's easy to nick yourself. Rinse off the razor every few strokes to keep it clean. Some women like to shave every day, others once or twice a week. It depends on individual hair growth.

Chemical Creams

Chemical creams remove leg hair down to the root. These creams should not be used under your arms because they can cause irritations and infections. Never use a product for your legs on your upper lip as it can cause serious irritation.

Waxing

Waxing removes hair by applying hot wax to the hair, covering the hair with gauze and allowing the wax to cool before pulling off the wax—and the hair with it. Many beauty salons give waxes or you can buy wax kits for your face, legs and swimsuit line at your local pharmacy.

Electrolysis

Electrolysis is a more permanent way of removing extreme cases of facial and leg hair. For most people, the hair does eventually grow back. The procedure, which uses an electrical current to destroy the hair root, should only be done by a trained technician.

Always read the manufacturer's instructions before using any product on your skin.

Facial Hair

Most all women have very fine hairs on their upper lip. If you have upper lip hair that is obviously dark or thick and bothers you, a cream or wax made especially for facial hair removal, may be used.

Bikini Line

Some styles of swimsuits call for the removal of some pubic hair. Because this area is extremely sensitive, removal should not be done by plucking hairs or by chemical removers. You can remove hair with special bikini wax kits or use a clean, sharp, disposable razor with shaving cream. Again, do a small area first to check for skin sensitivity.

Hair growth is an important external sign that you are maturing. I hope you enjoy these new changes

Hugs and kisses,
Mom

_____

_____

_____

_____

_____

_____

_____

_____

_____

Letter 6

Body Talk—Skin

Dear Larissa,

Skin, especially on our faces, is important to us. We want it to look good and feel good. During puberty, your skin may suffer due to hormonal changes in you body, stress, neglect, poor diet, or even illness. This letter explains some of the more common skin problems teens may have and some basic skin care techniques.

Acne

Acne is one body change that is bothersome for many teens. During puberty 79 percent of teens will be affected by skin problems: pimples (zits), whiteheads, blackheads, or acne.

Oil glands in your body produce an oily substance called sebum which keeps skin soft and supple. Unfortunately, these oil glands are especially numerous on your face, neck, shoulders, back, and upper chest. During puberty your oil glands work overtime producing more sebum than you need resulting in skin blemishes. A few teens experience little or no trouble with pimples, but the majority of teens have minor to major skin problems. Some teens have acne throughout their teenage years, others for only a year or two. A few people have acne into adulthood. If you experience acne, you are not alone. Most of the kids in your class share the same problem. Acne and the degree of its severity also tends to be hereditary. Teens whose parents had acne as teens will also likely have acne.

Wash your body's oily areas with a mild soap and water twice a day (morning and night), shampoo your hair frequently, wear clean clothes, and change clothes daily to help prevent new acne and clear up existing acne. Special anti-acne soaps and non-prescription acne medications are also available at your drugstore. For serious acne problems, our family doctor or a dermatologist can prescribe special medication. Watching your diet may also help. Some doctors think that greasy foods, candy and chocolate contribute to acne build-up.

Cold Sores (Fever Blisters)

Some teens are bothered by cold sores and cold sores aren't fun. When you're in school, a cold sore on your lip (much like a pimple on your chin) can feel like a huge blight on your face. You want it to heal as fast as possible.

Cold sores are caused by a type of herpes virus. Some people carry the virus in their bodies all their lives, while other people are not susceptible. The herpes cold sore virus is not the same herpes virus that gives people genital herpes. But, the virus is contagious. When you have a cold sore or you know of someone who does, don't exchange drinking glasses, handkerchiefs, eating utensils or kisses until the cold sore is healed. Once the virus is in your body, cold sores can break out at any time, especially if you're under stress or you have a cold or the flu. Mild cold sores can be treated with non-prescription medications. For severe cold sores, a doctor can prescribe stronger medication such as acyclovir.

Body Odor

During puberty, your sweat glands become more active, you perspire more, and have a stronger body odor. To keep body odor from being offensive to others take daily showers or baths and use either an underarm antiperspirant or underarm deodorant. Antiperspirants are designed to minimize perspiration. Deodorants cover or mask perspiration odor.

Wearing cotton clothing can also be helpful since cotton absorbs sweat better than synthetics. Because preteens are beginning puberty at earlier and earlier ages, some need deodorant or antiperspirant as early as fourth or fifth grade.

Here's a recap of basic adult hygiene.

- Wash oily areas of your body, your face, back, and arms at least twice a day.

- Medications and medicated soaps help fight acne.

- Wash your hair daily or at least every other day.

- Because adult body odor is strong, daily baths or showers are essential—including washing your genitals.

If you wear clean clothes, use deodorant or antiperspirant, and bathe or shower daily, you shouldn't have any problem with body odor. You'll feel clean and fresh, and more confident about yourself.

Here's to your beautiful, healthy skin.

Take care,
Mom

_____

_____

_____

_____

_____

_____

_____

_____

_____

Letter 7

Genitals and Reproductive System

Dear Larissa

When you begin puberty, you may be comfortable with breast development, but not genital development. Genital anatomy can seem confusing because it's a part of your body that you probably haven't studied in great detail.

"There are so many names to remember. How does everything work? Since my urethra and vaginal openings are so close together, isn't it dirty down there? And this pubic hair!"

Yes, there are some new names to learn. Unclean? If you bathe daily your genitals actually house fewer germs than your mouth.

Your outside genital area (vulva) includes your pubic hair, mons, clitoris, major and minor labia (lips), vaginal, and urethra openings. As you read this, you may want to use a mirror to locate each body part.

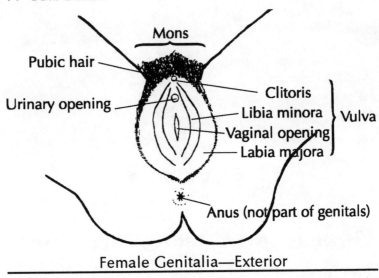

Female Genitalia—Exterior

Mons

Your mons is the pad of fatty tissue covering your pubic bone on which your pubic hair grows. Moving down, your mons divides into two separate sets of skin folds called labia majora (outside labia) and labia minora (inside labia). Labia is Latin for lips. Your labia are coverings for the clitoris and the vaginal and urinary openings. Labia are initially small and smooth. During puberty and through adulthood they become fleshier, wrinkly and darker in color.

Clitoris

Your clitoris is a small but highly, touch-sensitive bundle of nerves and tissue tucked under the end of your mons where your labia majora begins. It feels like a small knot. When massaged it is the female's most intense area of pleasurable, sexual feelings.

Orgasm (slang: climax, coming) is the pleasurable feeling you have when your clitoris has been rubbed to a release point of nerve stimulation. Orgasm is one of your body's natural sensory responses. Females most often experience orgasm through partner stimulation, intercourse, or masturbation.

Masturbation (self-touching) is a private way for people to become comfortable with their bodies, experience orgasm, and release sexual tension. For teens, masturbation is a healthy way to release sexual tension without having intercourse and risking pregnancy.

Most people masturbate. However some people feel uncomfortable touching themselves in this way, and a few religious orders prohibit masturbation. You decide what is right for you. You're normal if you do or don't. Although males don't have clitorises, they also masturbate and have orgasms. I'll explain how in my next letter.

Babies and young children often discover masturbation by accident when exploring their bodies, then forget about it until sometime during puberty. A female generally masturbates by rubbing her clitoris with her fingers, but vibrators are also sometimes used. Some women can experience orgasm during intercourse without manual stimulation of the clitoris; but other women need some type of manual stimulation by their partner or themselves before or during intercourse to achieve orgasm.

Reproductive System

Your reproductive system (internal sex organs) is nature's way for you to create and grow new life. The system consists of your ovaries, fallopian tubes, uterus, cervix, and vagina (see illustration on next page).

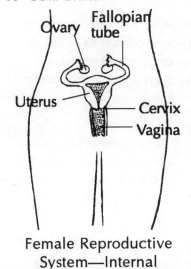

Female Reproductive
System—Internal

When your body begins functioning as an adult body, usually between ages nine and sixteen, you begin ovulation. Ovulation is a monthly cycle during which ova (eggs) in your ovaries begin to mature so they can be fertilized by male sperm to create new life. If the ovum (egg) is not fertilized by male sperm, the egg and the blood-rich bed prepared for it in your uterus dissolve and you menstruate (get your period). If the egg is fertilized, it attaches to the lining of your uterus where, if the conditions are right, the egg develops and grows into a baby. (See Letter 10, Conception and Pregnancy.)

Ovaries

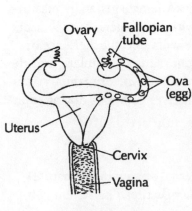

Route of the Egg

Ovulation (the monthly menstrual cycle) begins in your ovaries (see Letter 9, Menstruation). Your pituitary gland (an information center in your brain) sends a message (hormone) to either one of your ovaries to begin ripening an ovum. Normally one ovum matures each month and if the ovum is not fertilized you have your period.

When you're fully-grown your ovaries will be about the size of a thumb nail and contain all the ova you need for life. Females are born with ova—thousands of immature eggs of which only 400-500 will ever be released.

Fallopian Tubes

When the ovum is mature, it bursts from your ovary and is swept up by the tiny hairs on the ends of your fallopian tubes. Once in the fallopian tubes—which are no bigger than a string of spaghetti—the ovum makes a four-day journey to reach your uterus.

Uterus

When the egg reaches your uterus (womb), the uterus goes into action. If the egg is unfertilized, the egg and the endometrium (blood-rich lining of the uterus) dissolve and you get your period. The blood, anywhere from one tablespoon to a cup, is released through your cervix and travels out your vagina for three to seven days. For most women the menstruation process occurs monthly unless a woman is pregnant or nursing, has menstrual complications, has had a hysterectomy, or has completed menopause.

If the egg is fertilized, it attaches itself to the uterus. When you're fully grown, your uterus is only about the size of your fist. During pregnancy the uterus expands up to ten times its normal size to house and protect a baby (usually weighing seven to nine pounds at birth). After childbirth, it contracts back to its original size.

Cervix

The cervix is the lower part of your uterus that protrudes into the vagina. It has a tiny opening, the os, through which male sperm swim into your uterus. During childbirth the os and vagina expand wide enough to allow a

baby to pass through. When you are pregnant, a small mucus plug forms in the os to protect your baby from outside
infections. If you stick your finger toward the back of your
vagina, you can feel the end of your cervix and the os.

Vagina

Your vagina is a passageway of strong, elastic muscle that
leads to the uterus from outside your body. Stick a clean
finger in your vagina and feel its shape and texture. When
it's fully developed, your vagina is about three to five
inches long. Its an amazing muscle. The vagina is small
enough to hold a tampon in place to soak up menstrual
flow, yet it can expand large enough during childbirth to allow a baby to pass through. The vagina is where the male
inserts his penis during vaginal intercourse.

Since the vagina is the gateway to your reproductive organs
it's vital that your vagina be kept infection free. Otherwise
infections, especially sexually transmitted diseases (STDs),
can travel into your reproductive organs and damage them
enough to make you temporarily infertile or permanently
sterile (unable to have children).

Normally the vagina is irritation and infection free because
it cleans out impurities with its own acidic vaginal fluid.
Vaginal infections usually don't occur until a girl begins
menstruating. But once you begin your periods, anytime
your vagina contracts an infection it can't handle, you need
to seek medical treatment immediately. Symptoms of a
vaginal infection are normally itching or burning of the vagina, soreness, irritation, or swelling of the vulva and discomfort when urinating.

Wiping yourself incorrectly after a bowel movement, contracting a STD, having an allergic reaction to a contracep-

tive cream, foam, suppository or jelly, having several different sexual partners within a short time period, antibiotics, birth control pills, pregnancy, or diabetes can cause vaginal infections.

Common vaginitis (yeast infection) is a recurring, nuisance inflammation many women suffer from when the acidity level in their vaginal fluid drops, allowing normal vaginal yeast to grow out of control. For some women, foods high in sugar or yeast affect their acidity levels. If you experience vaginal burning or itching or if you insert your finger into your vagina and there is a cottage-cheese like residue on your finger you could have vaginitis. It is important that vaginitis be treated. If you ever experience these symptoms please tell me. Some doctors believe that untreated yeast infection can also infect other body systems. If non-prescription creams and suppositories don't clear up your symptoms, you should see a doctor. Yeast infection is very common. It's nothing to be embarrassed about because many women share the same affliction. Treating yeast infections should be a part of routine body care. If you aren't bothered by vaginitis, good for you.

Some STDs and vaginitis symptoms are similar and it's easy to mistake a STD for vaginitis and vice versa. Later, when you become sexually active ask your doctor about the similarities and differences between STDs and vaginitis symptoms.

In earlier times, some doctors advised women to clean their vaginas by douching—flushing their vaginas with water, water-vinegar, or commercial solutions. That's why companies still sell douches. But doctors today know that a woman's vagina is self-cleaning. Consistent douching may actually promote infections and rob your vagina of it's self-cleansing abilities. Unless a doctor prescribes douching with medication to treat an infection, douching is not recommended.

Hymen

When you explore your vagina with your finger, you may encounter your hymen. The hymen (slang: cherry, maidenhead) is a thin piece of skin that usually covers part or all of your vaginal opening. Some hymens are so small they're not noticeable and some women are born without hymens. Your hymen can be a solid covering with one big hole in it, many small holes, or it may be a thin fringe of skin around the outside of the opening.

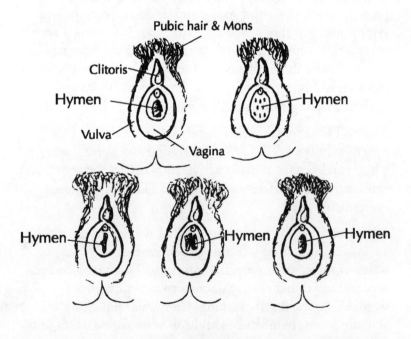

Hymen Varieties

In the old days, it was thought that every female had a solid hymen. If there was no blood from the hymen tear on the bed sheets, on the wedding night, it was believed that the bride wasn't a virgin (person who has not had intercourse) before she married. Today we know that not all females have solid hymens, and a hymen can be stretched or broken by tampons or vigorous exercise without intercourse taking place. Anyway, it's no one's business but you and your husband's whether both of you are or aren't virgins when you marry.

When your hymen is first stretched or torn by tampons, exercise, or intercourse, it may hurt and bleed a lot, a little, or not at all. But after the first complete tearing or stretching, any discomfort should disappear. If your hymen bleeds excessively or you have extreme pain—but rarely does that happen—let me know and we'll take you to see a doctor.

Larissa, your external sex organs and internal reproductive system are what allow you as an adult to have children. I know you will take good care of your body.

Mom

_____

_____

_____

_____

_____

_____

_____

_____

Letter 8

Urinary and Intestinal Systems

Dear Larissa,

As you are beginning to see, your body is a complicated mechanism with many interrelated parts. While the urinary and intestinal systems are not part of your reproductive system, they perform important bodily functions, and you should know about them.

Anatomically, your intestinal system actually starts with your mouth and includes your esophagus, stomach, large and small intestines, rectum and anus. Now, we're only concerned with the abdominal area. Your small and large intestines (bowels) break down solid wastes (feces, slang: poop) which are expelled out your anus.

Your urinary system begins with the bladder collecting and breaking down liquid wastes and expelling them as urine (slang: pee) through the urethra.

Though your reproductive, intestinal, and urinary openings are located close together, the three are distinctly separate (see the illustration below). Your anus expels solid
wastes. Your urethra expels urine. Blood flow during menstruation comes from your vagina.

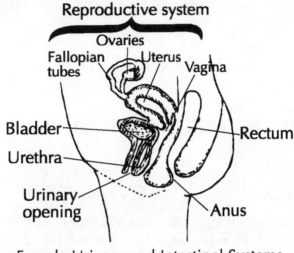

Female Urinary and Intestinal Systems

Although some people are susceptible to urinary and intestinal infections, the bladder and intestines usually function
smoothly. Good hygiene can help prevent potential problems.

♦ Wash your anal and urinary openings daily when you
    shower or bathe.

♦ Wear all-cotton or cotton crotch underwear. Synthet-
    ics can cause irritation by trapping bacteria in the
    genital area. Cotton lets your body breathe.

♦ After a bowel movement, clean your anus with toilet
    paper wiping backward instead of forward. Feces con-

taminated toilet paper brought forward over your vaginal and urinary openings can deposit bacteria that may cause irritations or infections.

♦ Anytime you notice blood in your stools or pain when urinating or having a bowel movement, tell me immediately so we can have it checked out. Irritations should be cleared up as quickly as possible so they don't turn into problem infections.

My next letter to you is about menstruation. Getting a period is one of the major changes in girls which can make them feel closer to becoming a woman.

Love,
Mom

_____

_____

_____

_____

_____

_____

_____

_____

_____

_____

LETTER 9

MENSTRUATION

Dear Larissa,

Getting your periods can be exciting or awkward until you become comfortable with the routine.

"This is what all my friends at school have talked about! Now I finally get my period and I feel self-conscious. Will everyone at school know I'm having my period? Will the guy I like know? What if he finds out? I'd be embarrassed. What if I start my period at school? Can people tell I'm having my period?"

I have one word to help you to deal with your monthly periods: *Relax.* The best way to handle your monthly period is to keep doing everything you normally do: sports, school activities, swimming, anything that doesn't cause you discomfort. You can begin ovulating as early as eight-years-old and continue until you are forty-five to fifty-five-years-old, but with the variety of sanitary products available today, no one needs to know you're having your period unless you choose to tell them.

Monthly periods are a part of being female. You may feel tired a day or two, experience mild cramps, a stomach ache, breast tenderness, feel bloated, or feel somewhat grumpy, but unless you suffer from severe cramps, severe depression, or true PMS (premenstrual syndrome) your period need not slow you down.

If you are feeling "blah," sympathetic words from a friend can help you beat the blahs. Your friend knows exactly how you're feeling and next week you can comfort her when she's having her period.

Exercises can help relieve menstrual cramps. Also, massaging your abdomen sometimes works, as well as placing a heating pad or hot-water bottle on your abdomen or lower back and taking aspirin or other pain relievers.

If you have bad cramps or headaches or a significant loss of energy, you may feel you need to scale back your activities for a few days each month. That's fine. Some women feel a definite loss of energy a few days each month, either during ovulation, before, or during their periods.

If you have severe cramps, you should see a doctor. Women who have extremely severe cramps may require prescription medication to help relieve the pain, or birth control pills to regulate the cycle.

Age of Onset

Girls normally start menstruating between eleven and seventeen years of age. Many girls begin sometime after their body weight reaches 100 pounds. However, this weight factor doesn't apply to small, petite girls or tall girls of slim build. Girls may experience a light, vaginal discharge, visible on their underpants a month or so before they get their periods.

Menopause

Women continue to menstruate until they stop ovulating normally between forty-five and fifty-five years of age. The ending of ovulation is called menopause. It can happen quickly or over a period of months or years. During this change women may experience hot flashes—seconds or minutes of feeling hot and heavily perspiring. Most women don't need medication unless hormone imbalances or other factors make menopause physically or emotionally painful. Menopause does not mean a woman's sex life is over. Unless we develop serious health problems, our sexuality is a part of us until we die.

Monthly Cycle

Your period comes in monthly cycles or menstrual cycles. A cycle is the time from the first day of bleeding of one period to the first day of bleeding of the next period. The average menstrual cycle is about twenty-eight days, but cycles can range from twenty-one days to thirty-five days. To

SUN	MON	TUE	WED	THU	FRI	SAT
		1	2	3	4	5
6	7	8	9	10	11	12
13	14	15	16	17	18	19
20	21	22	23	24	25	26
27	28	29	30	31		

Charting Your Period

keep track of your periods chart the days on a calendar.
That way, you'll have an idea when to expect your next one.

Missed Periods

In the beginning, it's not uncommon to have a period,
have one two weeks later, or miss a few months between periods. If you miss several months when you first begin menstruating and there is no reason to suspect pregnancy, don't
panic. Within a year your reproductive system should settle
into a somewhat predictable menstrual cycle, or you may
be a woman who only has periods once every three or six
months—and that will be normal for you.

Missed periods are cause for concern if you've had intercourse and you think you may be pregnant. But worry,
stress, and strenuous physical activity can also delay your
period—and stress seems to be a constant factor in our
lives today. The rule is: if you miss a period and you're concerned, talk to me about it.

Length of Period/Blood Flow

Just as the length of women's cycles vary, so does the dura-
tion and amount of bleeding. The average bleeding cycle is
five days, though periods can range from two to seven
days. Blood flow may range from one tablespoon to one
cup per period. The blood is actually a mixture of blood
and tissue. The flow can be smooth or clotted and bright
red to brown in color. Once your body establishes a length
and amount of blood flow, let me know if you experience
any changes and we'll discuss it with a doctor.

Bathing During Your Period

It's important when you're having your period to continue
taking your daily shower or bath and to wash your genital

area. Bathing washes away odor, helps prevent vaginal irritations, and helps you feel clean and fresh.

Spotting

Some women "spot" between their periods, that is, they have a day or two of very light bleeding, usually around the time they're ovulating. Spotting during ovulation is normal and can be taken care of by wearing a mini-pad or panty liner. However, unusual bleeding between periods should be checked by a doctor. Spotting and other menstrual irregularities are usually not serious, but whenever you have questions or uncertainties, don't hesitate to ask me or our doctor. Being in tune with your body's regular cycle means you can recognize a small abnormality before it has the chance to develop into something serious.

Be Prepared for Your First Period

Getting your first period will be a new experience, with a wide range of feelings. If you begin your period at home, you'll have supplies and the privacy of the bathroom. You'll also have some time to yourself to become used to the fact that you've started menstruating.

Many girls, though, start at school or in other public places. If there is a dispensing machine in a public bathroom, you shouldn't have any trouble obtaining a tampon or pad for yourself. If you're at school and you don't have a tampon or pad with you, you can ask the school nurse, a trusted teacher, or a friend for one.

When you start your period, you may notice a feeling of wetness. If there are only droplets of blood on your underwear, you can put on your pad or insert your tampon, and go on with your day. If no pad or tampon is available, a folded paper towel may work until you get home.

If you didn't realize you had started and blood has soaked through your clothes, call me. I will either pick you up so you can change clothes or make other arrangements for you. You may also be able to ask for help from a female teacher you are comfortable with, the school nurse, or a good friend who may have an extra pair of jeans or a skirt in her locker.

Since you will never know the exact time or where you'll start your first period, it's wise to always carry a sanitary pad (napkin) or tampon with you. I started in the seventh grade; you may start earlier or later. Some girls carry supplies with them a whole year before they actually start.

Tampons and pads are made of soft absorbent cotton and both work well soaking up menstrual flow. Some women prefer pads, others prefer tampons. Many girls begin with pads and later switch to tampons. You'll have to decide which is right for you.

Pads and tampons are wrapped in plastic wrappers or discreet carrying pouches that you can tuck into a zippered compartment in your purse or book bag. No one will know you're carrying them. I carry a tampon in my purse all the time.

You can usually buy menstrual supplies from dispensers in the school rest room and other public rest rooms. But beware; you'll need the correct change and occasionally you'll find machines empty or not working.

Tampons

A tampon is a small compressed cylinder of absorbent material that is inserted into the vagina to absorb the menstrual blood. Tampons come with plastic, cardboard, stick applicators or no applicator (you insert the tampon with your finger). You may want to try different brands of tampons to find which you like best. When properly inserted, your vagina holds the tampon in place so you can't feel it.

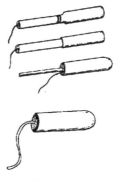

Tampons

Since a tampon is inserted into the body, during sports and other physical activities it won't hinder your activity like a bulky pad or napkin. Many women find tampons more comfortable than pads. Some women prefer pads. If you swim during your period, you must wear a tampon. A pad would become wet and leak blood into the pool.

Different blood flows require different sizes of tampons. Tampons are available in slim, junior, regular and super sizes. At first you'll want to use a junior or slim size. It was once thought that young girls shouldn't wear tampons because of a tendency toward bacteria build-up, but most doctors today don't feel there is any danger as long as you change your tampon regularly.

Always be sure to remove the last tampon when your period is finished. Because you can't feel the tampon it's easy to forget you're wearing one. Failing to change your tampons regularly puts you at a risk for a serious and sometimes fatal infection called TSS, (Toxic Shock Syndrome).

All tampon boxes have toxic shock syndrome warnings on the outside of the box. Read these warnings carefully. Report warning signs such as a fever, chills, vomiting, itching, irritation of the genitals, or persistent unpleasant odor or unusual discharge from the vagina to me or our doctor immediately. Tampons have been used since Egyptian times and they are normally very safe; but severe and untreated TSS can kill.

Insertion

When using a tampon with an applicator, first work the applicator in your hands to see how the applicator operates. Then throw that tampon and applicator in the trash and take out a new unit.

Never insert a tampon and applicator that have been dropped on the floor. It may have picked up dirt, lint, and germs from the floor. To avoid infections only clean tampons should be inserted into the vagina.

If your hymen is fully intact, you may have to gently stretch your hymen with your finger for a couple of months before you can use a tampon. Start with a junior or slim size. Before insertion carefully read the instructions. Tampons can be inserted standing up, lying down, or sitting on the toilet. I like sitting on the toilet. You may prefer another position.

When inserting the tampon, angle the tampon toward the small of your back because that is how your vagina is positioned. If you don't angle the tampon you'll hit your vaginal walls making insertion difficult. When you're learning to insert tampons, you may not get the first one inserted correctly. Take it out, and begin again with a new tampon. Keep repeating the process until the tampon feels comfortable and is fully inside the vagina.

To insert the tampon, you may have to part your labia to reach the vaginal opening. Relax. If you're tense, the vaginal opening will contract, making insertion difficult. If your vagina is naturally dry, you can lubricate your tampon with K-Y jelly purchased at our local pharmacy. Do not use lotion or face cream to lubricate the tampon; they may contain chemicals which could irritate your vagina.

A girlfriend of mine didn't read the tampon instructions and used up a whole box of tampons learning to insert one correctly. Her mom thought she'd had quite a first period until my friend told her mom what had happened. But if it takes using a dozen tampons to learn proper insertion, that's what you need to do.

You shouldn't be able to feel an inserted tampon except for the string coming out of your vagina. If you can feel your tampon it isn't pushed in far enough. You can try pushing it further into your vagina with a clean finger, or you may have to pull it out and insert a new tampon.

There is no chance of a tampon getting lost inside your body because the cervix opening is about the size of the head of a pin and your tampon has no place to go. Do make sure the end of the string is hanging from your vagina, so you can remove the tampon for your next tampon change.

A correctly inserted tampon won't fall out because the muscles inside the vagina hold it secure. The only exception to this is that occasionally the muscles you use in having a bowel movement may cause your tampon to move downward. To correct this, after properly wiping yourself, take a clean finger and gently push your tampon back into place.

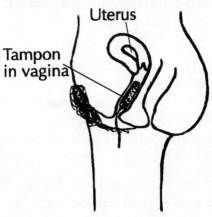

Uterus

Tampon in vagina

Tampon Inserted in the Vagina

When a tampon is fully absorbed with blood, leakage may occur onto your underpants. To prevent stains, you may want to wear a mini pad on the days of your heaviest blood flow.

If tampon use seems complicated or insertion is difficult, you can use sanitary pads or napkins. The choice is yours.

Changing and Disposing of Tampons

Tampons should be changed every three or four hours to prevent bacteria build-up and leakage. Tampons should be wrapped in toilet paper and put in our bathroom wastebasket. In public rest rooms, wrap the tampon and put it in the sanitary disposal container in the stall or in the rest room trash can.

Although most tampon companies advertise flushable tampons, it's a good idea to never flush tampons, their applicators or sanitary pads down the toilet. They can seriously clog plumbing, causing backups and costly repair bills.

Sanitary Pads or Napkins

Sanitary pads or napkins are the other most popular way to collect menstrual flow. Pads and napkins are available in different sizes and thicknesses for the light, medium, or heavy blood flows. Maxi pads are for medium to heavy flow. Mini pads are for light flow. Pads or napkins are made of layers of soft cotton or other absorbent material and most of them are made with a plastic lining. Some are made with fold-over "wings" to prevent blood from staining your underwear.

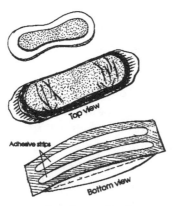

Sanitary Pad

Wearing a Pad

The most popular sanitary pads have adhesive strips so you can press the napkin onto the inside crotch of your underpants. Some pads are made to be held in place by a sanitary belt worn around your waist. You can also pin a pad to your underpants with safety pins.

Wearing pads usually feels awkward at first—especially the thicker pads. Though it might seem to you that people can tell you're wearing a pad, check yourself in a mirror—the pad doesn't show. Once you get used to wearing pads, you can participate in about any sport, except swimming.

Changing and Disposing of Pads

Like tampons, pads and napkins should be changed every three or four hours, wrapped in toilet paper and disposed of in a waste can or sanitary receptacle. Flushing pads down the toilet can be even worse than tampons for clogging plumbing.

Regular changes are necessary to avoid blood soaking through the pad and to prevent odor. Menstrual blood is odorless until it comes in contact with germs in the air and vagina. Changing pads prevents odor.

Getting your period is a big event. If you feel like celebrating, we can order pizza or go to a movie. If you want some quiet time alone, or with a girlfriend, that's fine, too. Most females feel somewhat overwhelmed during their first few periods. I hated getting my period because I was athletic. To me it was a bother; you may look forward to getting your period. Both feelings are normal.

Mom, why do girls have to deal with monthly periods and pregnancy and guys don't? It doesn't seem fair.

I didn't think it was fair either, Larissa—until I had you. You have to consider the fact that although guys don't have periods, they can't have babies, either. Even though I don't know any woman who likes having periods, menstruating means you can someday have children of your own. Having the ability to give birth to you is one of the reasons I'm glad I'm female.

Love,
Mom

_____

_____

_____

_____

_____

_____

_____

_____

_____

_____

Letter 10

Conception and Pregnancy

Dear Larissa,

Parents and teens often find the topics of conception and pregnancy the most difficult to discuss. In some cases, parents today may not even know the correct information because their parents never knew or communicated it to them. I hope this letter gives you a solid understanding of the subject.

As you may know from health class, human conception—the creation of new life—normally happens through intercourse (slang: having sex, doing it, making love, messing with). You may wonder how intercourse works and what it feels like.

Pre-teens often find the idea of intercourse gross. They wonder if their parents still "do it." If two people are relaxed and feel comfortable with each other, intercourse can be a pleasurable, loving activity they can enjoy even into their seventies, eighties, and nineties. Below is an illustration of the erect penis inside the vagina.

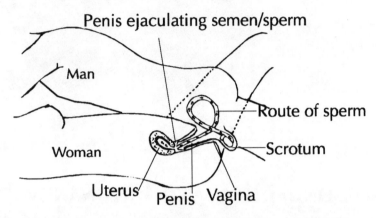

Penis ejaculating semen/sperm

Man

Route of sperm

Woman

Scrotum

Uterus   Penis   Vagina

During intercourse the male's penis becomes erect (hard), and he inserts it into the female's vagina and releases semen and sperm. Semen is a sticky white liquid containing sperm (the male reproductive cell). Sperm are so small that more than 300,000,000 sperm can be released into the vagina in one ejaculation, and it takes only one of those sperm for you to become pregnant. Unless you're planning a family, you should never have sex without birth control—just remember the 300,000,000 sperm in each ejaculation swimming toward your one ovum.

After ejaculation, sperm in the semen immediately begin swimming toward the top of the vagina, through the cervix and uterus, and into the fallopian tubes looking for an egg to fertilize. If they don't find an ovum, they die. Sperm that don't make the swim to the fallopian tubes fall back into the semen which trickles down the vagina and out of the woman's body. They too die.

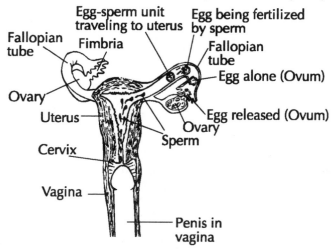

Sperm's Trip From Penis to Fertilize Ovum

But, sperm can live in the uterus and fallopian tubes up to three days before dying so it's easy to become pregnant. For conception to occur it only takes one sperm out of the millions ejaculated to find a ripe ovum and penetrate it.

After conception the fertilized egg travels down the fallopian tube into the uterus where it attaches itself to the uterine wall. Once attached, if the egg is allowed to develop, it will grow into a baby.

Occasionally the body naturally aborts (miscarries) the pregnancy. Doctors suspect miscarriages occur because the fertilized ovum was defective in some way or your body was not ready to sustain the pregnancy.

Imprinted in a fertilized ovum are twenty-three pairs of chromosomes plus one X and one X or Y chromosome—representing the exact blueprint of how we will develop: our hair color, height, weight. . .everything. It is a miracle how one ovum and one sperm, when united can become a wailing eight pound little person in nine months.

Pregnancy

A full-term pregnancy is approximately 280 days long (forty weeks or nine full lunar months). For the first forty-eight hours the developing fertilized egg is called a zygote. When the egg attaches itself to the uterus, it is an embryo. At eight weeks human features become apparent and the developing life is called a fetus. The fetus then develops into a baby.

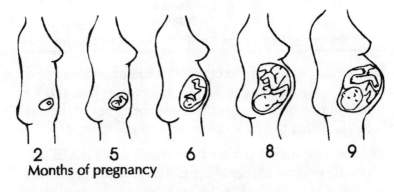

2   5   6   8   9
Months of pregnancy

Fetal Development

Becoming Pregnant

There are a few days during ovulation (your monthly menstrual cycle) that are optimum times for conception. But due to stress, diet and infections your ovulation cycle can vary monthly. Not being able to accurately pinpoint your ovulation and the length of time sperm can live in the fallopian tubes, is why it's possible for you to conceive anytime during your menstrual cycle. The first signs that you are pregnant may be nausea, vomiting, tender breasts and a missed period.

The Pregnancy

The first three months (first trimester) of pregnancy most women experience mild-to-severe morning sickness (nausea and for some women vomiting). This is your body's reaction to the new changes going on inside. You usually also feel tired and need extra sleep. I was pretty sick the first three months during the pregnancies for you and your brother.

To assure that the early pregnancy is progressing normally, you need to visit the doctor and she or he will put you on a regular schedule of visits. Eliminate smoking, drinking alcohol, and all other drugs unless prescribed by the doctor.

During the middle stage of pregnancy (second trimester) you'll usually regain your energy and feel the best you'll feel throughout the pregnancy. I felt good the second trimester; but the third trimester was not so easy.

In the last trimester your wrists and joints will probably swell from extra body fluid. Heartburn is common because your internal organs are all compressed and pushed out of position to make room for the baby. The baby's pressure on your bladder causes you to constantly have to urinate. Carrying the baby is exhausting. When you look down, your belly is so full of baby you can't see your feet. In the last month you feel sluggish and heavy and wonder if your delivery date will ever arrive.

Imagine what it would be like if you're a teen and you have to go to school and keep up your grades, feeling like this. The stress pregnancy places on a teen's still developing body is enormous and not healthy.

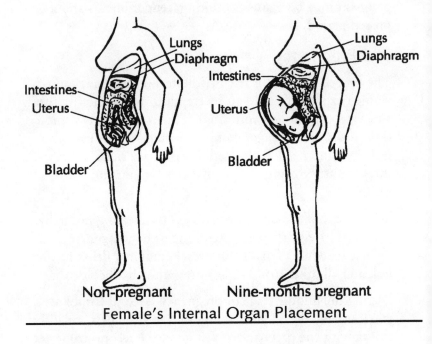

Non-pregnant   Nine-months pregnant

Female's Internal Organ Placement

Childbirth

Childbirth is hard work for you and the baby. At the end of the ninth month, when the baby is ready to be born, your uterus begins to contract and you go into labor. During labor the uterine muscles gradually build strength and the cervix and vaginal canal dilate (open) so the baby can be pushed out of the vaginal canal and into the world.

Labor and childbirth are painful. The pain ranges from moderate to extreme. Once the baby is born the immediate delivery pain is over although some women also experience post-delivery discomfort. The average length of labor for first deliveries is twelve to fourteen hours; seven hours for succeeding births.

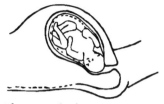

1. The cervix is
   fully dilated

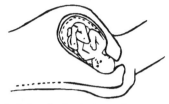

2. The baby's head
   moves into the vagina

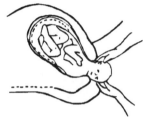

3. The baby's head
   comes out of vagina

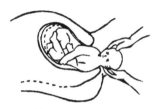

4. The baby's
   shoulders follow

Childbirth and Delivery

Some Final Thoughts

As a developing teen you are a sexual person. Around age twelve to fourteen most people become aware of their sex drive. All people have a sex drive—it makes us want to be touched, loved and cared about. Because your growth hormones are working overtime during adolescence, your sexual feelings can be intense. Being with a special person feels good. Touching is nice. You like to date, but you don't want to become pregnant or contract a STD. What do you do?

When you begin dating and going together, you will need to make some adult decisions about how to manage the sexual feelings you have. What is right and wrong in dating? What is going too far? What sexual activities put you at risk for pregnancy and diseases? These issues we'll talk about in the next few letters. How do you feel about teen pregnancy and having sex?

This letter contains an enormous amount of information. It's information you need to know and information you can reread as your body continues to develop. If there is anything you don't understand or if you have any questions, ask me anytime.

Thanks, Mom. everything in this letter is good information. but what about boys and dating? When are we going to talk about guys?

Okay Larissa, that's what my next letters are all about. Keep reading.

Mom

_____

_____

_____

_____

_____

_____

_____

_____

_____

LETTER 11

WHAT YOU SHOULD KNOW
ABOUT GUYS' BODIES

Dear Larissa,

Larissa, while you're developing and changing, so are the
guys in your class. I remember in seventh grade seeing my
first picture of a naked man. The rest of the year I sat in
class stealing glances at the boys, wondering if they all
looked like the picture.

Because it takes male sperm to make a female pregnant,
you need to know how the male body functions. The illustrations on the next few pages detail male puberty growth
and describe how the male reproductive system works.
Guys experience physical and emotional changes also. I'll
tell you about some of these in this letter. Testosterone is
the main male hormone responsible for body development.

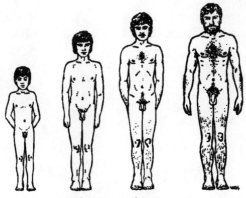

Male Development

Chest

Of course guys don't develop breasts like we do, but as they mature their chests do broaden and become more muscular. During male development the area around a guy's nipples may appear fleshy—almost like stage one of female breast development. The swelling, called gynecomastia, usually disappears within a year. However overweight males may always have fleshy chests. Guys are usually sensitive about having a fleshy chest and don't like to be teased about it anymore than we like being teased about our periods or developing breasts.

Voice

Unlike girls, guys' voices become deeper in tone as they go through puberty. The reason is that male vocal cords mature differently than female vocal cords.

Pubic Hair

Males also go through five stages of pubic hair growth. They may begin hair growth as early as nine years of age or as late as sixteen. Hair begins growing around the base of the penis, onto the scrotum and upwards toward the belly-button (navel). Male pubic hair is like ours in that it begins with a few slightly curly hairs and becomes a mass of darker, tight curls. It, too, is there to protect sensitive genital areas.

Body Hair

Males grow hair under their arms, on their chests, legs, and sometimes even on the tops of their hands. But unlike us, guys grow facial hair. They can shave daily or grow a beard or mustache. Male hair growth is hereditary. Some men have very hairy chests, arms, legs and faces and other men don't have much hair at all. Some men even grow hair on their backs.

Male Genital Anatomy

The male exterior genitals include the penis, glans (tip of the penis), scrotum (houses the testicles) and urethral opening.

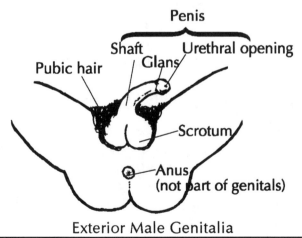

Exterior Male Genitalia

The anus (although shown here, is not part of the reproductive system) is the same in both females and males and dispels solid wastes from the large and small intestines.

Penis and Urethra

The male penis is small when a guy is still a boy. When he starts puberty, the penis begins growing much the same as your vulva develops. The inside of the penis is made of spongy tissue with the urethra running down the middle of the penis. The male urethra serves a duel function and releases urine and sperm—but never at the same time.

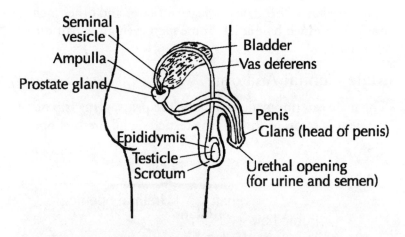

Seminal vesicle
Ampulla
Prostate gland
Bladder
Vas deferens
Penis
Glans (head of penis)
Epididymis
Testicle
Scrotum
Urethal opening
(for urine and semen)

Dual Urethra Function

The urethra is a hollow tube that runs down the middle of the penis and is connected to the bladder and to the vas deferens. When a male urinates, urine from the bladder travels through the urethra and out the urethra opening at the glans (the tip of the penis). When a male become sexually aroused and ejaculates (releases sperm and semen), a valve on the bladder automatically shuts off urine flow to allow semen flow.

Circumcision

Male penises can be circumcised or uncircumcised. Circumcision is a procedure where the sheath of skin (foreskin) covering the glans is cut away. The operation dates back to biblical days and was originally done to honor religious beliefs. Circumcision is usually done in the hospital within a day or so after a baby boy is born. There is some pain involved in the procedure.

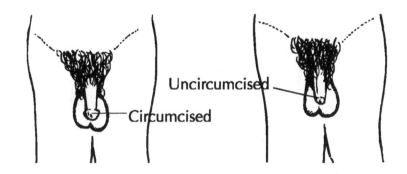

Uncircumcised

Circumcised

Circumcised and Uncircumcised Male Penis

Before the 1940s most males in America weren't circumcised. From the 1940s to the 1980s the medical community recommended circumcision for hygienic reasons. Doctors felt that circumcised penises were easier to clean and keep free from disease. Today circumcision is a choice left up to the parents. If the boy pulls the foreskin back and washes himself daily, infections shouldn't be a problem. Many parents still have their sons circumcised. Other parents elect not to circumcise. Circumcision does not affect sexual performance.

Erections

The male penis can be flaccid (empty) or erect (full). During an erection blood fills the penis' spongy tissue and the muscles at the penis base tighten so the blood stays in the penis. This makes the penis longer, thicker and firm. When the erection lessens, the blood flows back out the spongy tissue and the penis returns to its flaccid (empty) state.

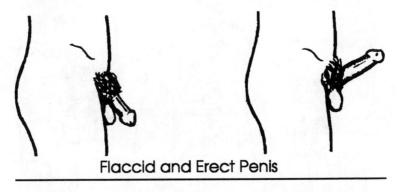

Flaccid and Erect Penis

An erection (slang: hard on, boner) is necessary for sexual intercourse. I'll talk about that shortly. Unfortunately, just as we can get our periods anytime males can get erections anytime, and that's embarrassing to them. Most commonly males can have erections if they are sexually aroused or thinking sexual thoughts. However, guys also get erections without being sexually excited or without the penis even being touched. Non-sexual erections are called "spontaneous" erections. During puberty guys can have spontaneous erections anytime—at school, at home or on a date. As one teen male told me, "guys feel self-conscious just like girls feel self-conscious."

"I'm a jock. I play basketball, football and run track. When my body started changing I acted cool, but I was actually very self-conscious. One day I was walking down the hall in school and I had an erection. I thought, What do I do now? I'm not even thinking about sex but everyone is going to notice this bulge in my jeans. All I can remember is that I held my books in front of me and prayed it would go away."

The best action to take if you notice that a guy is having an erection is to ignore it. Save the guy from embarrassment like you'd like him to ignore the situation if you start your period in class or your purse drops open and your tampons or pads fall out.

Penis Size

Male penis sizes varies like women's breast sizes vary. Average adult penis size is three to five inches long when flaccid (empty) and five to seven inches long when erect (full). Like female breast size, male penis size has nothing to do with what kind of person a guy is or what kind of friend, boyfriend, or husband he would be.

Interior Reproductive System

The male interior reproductive anatomy includes the testicles (testes), vas deferens, ampulla, prostate gland, Cowper's glands, and epididymis.

Testicles and scrotum

The testicles, where sperm are made, are encased in a sac called the scrotum (slang: balls) which hangs outside the body. Inside of the testes (testicles) are hundreds of tiny tubes call tubules which make millions of sperm daily. Males begin making sperm at the onset of puberty and keep making sperm until their sixties or older. Sperm that is not released through ejaculation is absorbed back into the body.

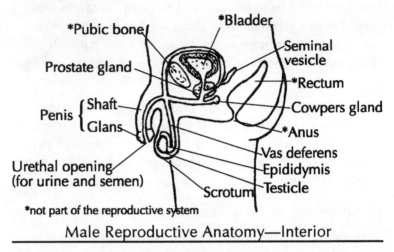

*Pubic bone

*Bladder

Prostate gland

Seminal vesicle

*Rectum

Penis { Shaft
Glans

Cowpers gland

*Anus

Urethal opening
(for urine and semen)

Vas deferens
Epididymis
Testicle

Scrotum

*not part of the reproductive system

Male Reproductive Anatomy—Interior

Epididymis, vas deferens, ampulla, prostate gland, Cowper's glands

After sperm are made in the testicles, they travel to the epididymis where they are stored for about six weeks while ripening. The sperm then travel through the vas deferens to the ampulla. The ampulla is a storage compartment attached to the seminal vesicles where the sperm are stored until ejaculation. The seminal vesicles produce the semen which is mixed with the sperm for ejaculation. The Cowper's glands secrete a fluid that cleanses the urethra before semen is released. When a male ejaculates (releases the semen), genital muscles helped by the prostate gland force the semen through the urethra and out the glans (head of the penis).

The male reproductive system is also complex like the female's. All anatomy must be in working order to produce healthy sperm.

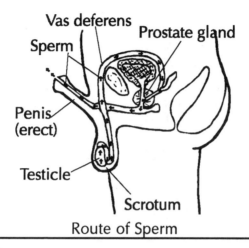

Route of Sperm

During puberty male growth hormones work overtime and cause males to produce a huge amount of sperm. The body must then release this sperm. Methods of release are through nocturnal emissions (wet dreams), masturbation, and intercourse.

Wet Dream/Nocturnal Emission

The wet dream is so named because it happens at night. While a guy is asleep, he has an erection and ejaculates. When he awakes, he finds one to two tablespoons of semen on his stomach or pajamas.

Most males have nocturnal emissions and these can begin for guys as early as age ten. A guy's first wet dream is as much a surprise to him as our periods are to us. Guys are usually as secretive about their wet dreams as we are about our periods. Neither girls or guys should tease each other about any of the body changes we experience during puberty.

Masturbation

Masturbation or self-touching is another way to release sperm build-up, but it's a private activity guys (and girls) usually don't want anyone knowing about. A guy masturbates by rubbing his penis until the muscles have been stimulated enough to force ejaculation. Masturbation is also much better than having intercourse and taking the chance of a girl becoming pregnant.

Sexual Intercourse

Intercourse is the third way for guys to release sperm build-up, but a guy must guard against contracting STDs and making a girl pregnant. Unless a guy is in a committed relationship and ready to handle the emotions and birth control responsibilities of intercourse, masturbation is a better choice than intercourse.

One story that is not true is that if a guy has an erection he must have sex or he'll suffer pain from "blue balls" (trapped semen). Erections will subside on their own and the semen will be expelled through the urine or absorbed back into the reproductive organs. A guy who has an erection, does not have to have intercourse.

Genital Hygiene

- To care for his genitals, a guy needs to wash his penis and scrotum daily when he showers or bathes. Guys who are uncircumcised must pull their foreskin back and wash the area thoroughly.

◆ Guys should always avoid direct hits to the genital area. A direct hit can render a guy unconscious and damage his testes.

That's why when guys are involved in sports they wear athletic supporters (jock straps) to hold the penis and testes close to the body to help avoid injury. There are two types of supporters: a cloth supporter for light contact sports and a plastic cup supporter for sports like baseball and football. Supporters comes in S-M-L sizing and are similar to bras in that they support the sexual anatomy and help protect it from damage and injury.

◆ Guys should also practice a weekly self-examination of their testicles. Testicular cancer is found in about four of every 100,000 white men each year. The rate is lower for males of other races. The cancer is most common between the ages of twenty and thirty-four but also occurs in younger and older men. Anytime a guy notices a change in his testicles, such as, enlargement of the testicle, small, hard lump on the testicle, or feeling of heaviness in a testicle he should see a doctor.

Mom, wait a second. This is all good information, but I think guys' penises are kind of gross. Right now, I like people with their clothes on better than off. Do people find genitals sexy?

Larissa, I didn't think guys' penises or my genitals were attractive in my teen years, either. As you reach adulthood, you may feel differently. For now, you don't have to worry about it.

What you do want to keep in mind is that once a guy and girl begin puberty, your bodies are capable of creating a pregnancy. Today, in cities around America, twelve and thirteen-year-olds are finding themselves pregnant. That's very sad for them, their families, and their babies. Having sex when dating is a serious responsibility. We'll talk about dating, sex, and love in my next few letters.

Take care,
Mom

_____

_____

_____

_____

_____

_____

_____

_____

_____

Letter 12

Dating—The Basics

Dear Larissa,

Why do people date? Why do girls like guys? Guys can be so weird. Why do guys like girls?

It's human nature. Male and female being together is as old as the world. You begin dating because there is something that attracts you to a person. The guy you like may have great eyes, a cute smile, a nice laugh or a muscular body. You may be attracted to him because he's funny, cool, serious or sexy. . . .

Sometimes you can't even describe why you like someone—it's just how you feel. Why did I like your father? Why did he like me?

Teens told me that once they are attracted to each other, they date for many reasons:

- They date to get to know each other.

- They date for fun.

- They date for romance.

- They date to feel grown-up.

- They date to find out what personality traits they like and dislike in people.

Later on people date to find a committed partner, for marriage and to raise children together.

Unfortunately, people also date for the wrong reasons, such as, dating for status or dating for sex. When you date someone because of his stature, you don't really care about the person. He may look good on your arm or give you a higher standing in school. Maybe he's dating you for the same reason. Other teens date to boost their self-esteem or in the hope of finding love and attention they aren't getting from parents. I'll talk more about dating relationships in Letter 13.

The most important reason to date is that dating helps you decide what you like and dislike in a person—you get to know a person. It also gives you experience dealing with relationships and teaches you what makes a relationship work. And, dating is usually fun.

Stages of Dating

There are generally three stages of dating in teen relationships.

Stage 1: Junior high/middle school

Normally, girls and guys start liking each other and "going together" in junior high or middle school. But because you can't drive yet, your time together is limited to school, after school, and school activities. Junior high "going together" is usually short-term dating because guys and girls aren't yet comfortable with dating. A guy may be brave one week and want to go together. The next week he'll get scared and break up. You may do the same thing. Opinions from friends also play a part in who you do and don't date. Opinions often change weekly shortening middle school relationships.

Stage 2: Freshman/sophomore years

During freshman and sophomore years of high school, girls continue to be interested in dating. High school relationships generally last longer than junior high dating, but long-term commitments (one or more years) aren't yet the norm. You're still learning about dating, your likes, and dislikes.

Some girls want to date older guys because they seem more mature. You may enjoy being with Brian, a junior, rather than freshman, Danny, who sits next to you in English. There is a problem for younger girls who date older guys.

Older guys may be more sexual and more sexually experienced. Some guys date younger girls for one reason only—the sex—and they always tell you they love you. They get sex and dump you; it's the oldest, meanest game in the book. Guys will keep doing it as long as we girls fall for it.

Have respect for yourself. Tell those guys to take a hike. They aren't worth the spit on the sidewalk. The one worry every parent has is that a daughter will be talked into having sex before she's ready, she won't use birth control, and she'll face a teen pregnancy.

Someday if you date an older guy, you want to make sure he's dating you for you and not for the sex. I dated an older guy when I was in high school. He was great but there were other guys in his class you couldn't trust. There will always be guys you can't trust just as there are some girls guys shouldn't trust.

Stage 3: Junior/senior years

By your junior and senior years of high school you may be:

- going with someone,

- you've had it with guys and you're hanging around with your girlfriends waiting for life after high school, or

- you have a group of guy and girl friends you do things with.

By your senior year you will have formed some opinions of what does and doesn't make a good date and a good relationship.

How do you know if a guy is worth dating or not? One way is the dolphin versus shark test. Dolphins are intelligent, gentle, and fun to be with. Sharks are sly, aggressive, selfish scavengers, who take whatever they can get. The same is true in dating. Some people are dolphins, others are sharks.

When you start liking a guy or he starts liking you, take a good look at the guy. See if he matches the shark list or the dolphin list. Go for the dolphins. Stay away from the sharks. Sharks are only out for themselves. They get what they want from a girl and dump her.

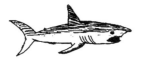

SHARKS	DOLPHINS
1. Big Egos	1. Intelligent
2. Aggressive	2. Kind
3. Deceiving	3. People Oriented
4. Sleek/polished	4. Pleasing appearance
5. Attack People	5. Helpers
6. Scavengers	6. Joiners
7. Selfish	7. Loving, Faithful
8. Dress Up In	8. Always Themselves
Dolphin's Clothes	

Mom, at what age can I date? How about car dating?

Larissa, each family has different guidelines for dating. Many families still adhere to fifteen or sixteen as a mature age to car date, but they allow their sons and daughters in middle school to meet friends at the movies, the mall or school activities. Then there is weekend dating versus school night dating. Most families want to meet the guys their daughters date. Since you asked when you can begin dating, we'll have to sit down and talk about it.

We will have to decide on a reasonable time for you to come home from your dates. I know home time, (often called a curfew) can seem like parents are being totally un-fair. But home time isn't a plot designed to keep you from having fun. Home time is a safeguard.

Larissa, I love you more than anything else in the world, even those times I forget to tell you. A parent's greatest fear when their teens begin car dating or riding in a car with friends to ball games and movies is that they'll be involved in a car accident and be hurt or killed.

Teens under age twenty rate the highest number of car accidental deaths in any age group. A teen dies in a car accident every eleven minutes. More than fifty percent of all traffic deaths involve a drunk driver or a driver on drugs. (Statistics, National Safety Council).

Home time is a safeguard to help protect you against drunk drivers and decrease the chance that you or a friend will fall asleep at the wheel and end up in a ditch. I loved going out with my friends when I was a teen. Looking back now, I'm glad my parents loved me enough to give me a home time, so I didn't end up dead.

But let's move on to more cheerful subjects. My next letter to you is a long one and it's chock full of all sorts of dating and relationship information. It's titled Dating, Relationships, and Friends. You can be sure it will be good reading.

I love you!
Mom

_____

_____

_____

_____

_____

_____

_____

Letter 13

Dating, Relationships, and Friends

Dear Larissa,

When a girl and a guy start dating or going together, they've entered into a relationship. From the time you start dating and you're involved with a guy, you will be in a relationship.

Relationship is defined in Webster's Dictionary as: the state of being "mutually" interested or involved with one another. Mutually means both the guy and girl like and care for each other.

Some people date because that's how they maintain self-esteem. They only know how to feel good about themselves through other people. Using dating for self-love is destructive. It's a false high that destroys self-worth. The greatest thing you can do for yourself is to love you for being you!

At times in your life you will wrestle with your self-esteem—everyone does. When something is troubling you, it's impossible to feel good. Talking to me or a close friend can often help. If you can't work out your dilemma with a friend's help, seek professional help from a counselor or psychologist.

The things that make you a neat person are your smile, sense of humor, honor, loyalty to friends, and caring attitude. Each of us is a beautiful person; we just don't realize it sometimes.

A relationship will not solve life's problems, but it should be a positive addition to your life. Here is a checklist of qualities a good relationship should have. Use it to evaluate whether a relationship is good.

+ You both feel good about dating each other. Neither of you is embarrassed to have people know that you are dating.

+ You can talk to each other and share private thoughts.

+ You have similar values and beliefs.

+ You respect each other. You focus on each other's good points rather than weaknesses.

+ You both care for and equally support each other.

+ You have interests together and apart from each other. You like being together, but you don't have to be with each other every minute of the day.

+ You may argue and disagree, but you can both laugh at your disagreements afterward.

* Your relationship is not verbally or physically abusive. Neither of you beat, hit, or yell at each other.

* You both realize that a relationship is compromise— each partner caring for the other partner's welfare.

For a relationship to have a chance, positive qualities must be evident within the first few meetings. Long-term relationships take time to develop—weeks, months, years.

The majority of middle school and high school dating is short-term when you're:

* Learning about relationships.

* Dating different people to find out what you like.

Relationship Situations

Teen relationships, like adult relationships, can be good, bad, and frustrating. The following are different situations most everyone has experienced at one time or another. I hope reading about them will help you in similar situations.

You like a guy but he isn't interested in you

This is an age-old problem. You like a guy, but he isn't interested in you. When you like someone but find out he's not interested in you, you may have feelings of disappointment, sadness, and frustration. You may put yourself down, thinking you're not interesting or pretty enough.

When I was in high school, I couldn't count the number of guys I wanted to date who weren't attracted to me. I'd get excited about a guy, and he didn't even know I existed. Have you had experiences like this?

If a guy isn't interested in you it means the two of you aren't meant to be together. There is someone else for you. Sometimes, it's impossible to believe there could be anyone else. But there is—and he's usually waiting around the next corner.

Getting a guy to like you

You can't. You simply can't. People are attracted to each other or they aren't. You can get a guy to notice you by spending time where he spends time or working on a project together, but you can't make another person like you. You only cause yourself disappointment and pain trying to make happen what isn't meant to be.

Telling a guy you are not interested in him

Larissa, telling someone "I like you as a person, but I'm not attracted to you as someone to date" can be very difficult. It's a conversation you may have many times in your life. The best way to tell someone is straight out in a firm, honest way, without making excuses and without putting them down. For example:

> "Rob, you're nice-looking and fun, but I'm not attracted to you as someone to date. I'd rather be truthful with you than make excuses. I'm sorry but us going out won't work."

When the time comes to tell a guy you aren't attracted to him, how do you think you'll say it?

Talking to your date

Communicating—listening and sharing—is the essence of relationships. Communicating is sharing yourself with another person. It can be the toughest job in the world. In dating (and marriage) it's always easier to kiss someone than to verbally tell them what that kiss means. Is that kiss friendship, like, love, or lust?

Communicating is tough because it's sharing your personality and inner feelings with someone. That's scary because that person may or may not accept you. But you have to take the risk. If you don't communicate, you don't have intimacy and you don't have a relationship—whether it's friendship or a dating relationship. The following suggestions may help.

- Take it slow. Ask the person out for a date. Talk about school, movies, music, sports, family, dreams, or goals. Listen to your date when he is talking. If you are shy and find it hard to talk, write down a list of things you could talk about. Practice talking in a mirror at home before you go out on the date. It may seem awkward practicing in a mirror, but it should help you feel more at ease—especially if he's a guy you really like. List some things you could talk about with someone.

- If you realize on the first date that you aren't right for each other, you can go your separate ways. You have each learned something about yourself. No harm done.

- If you both like the first date, be honest with each other about your feelings and make plans to go out again.

- Remember. You have to take a risk to develop any dating relationship or friendship.

Asking a guy out or telling a guy you like him

In a national poll, the majority of high school guys surveyed said they wanted girls to ask them out. Today it's okay for girls to ask guys out. The best way to ask someone out is to give him a call or talk to him at school. If you are shy, ask a trusted friend to let the guy know you are interested in him.

When a guy turns you down for a date

This is rejection and guys have been rejected by girls for years. No wonder guys are so shy when asking girls out. Being turned down hurts. Not everyone you like is going to like you.

You really wanted to go out with this guy. He turned you down. You're hurt or embarrassed. You want to avoid him. That's okay. After a turn down everyone needs time to muster their self-esteem again. Guys feel the same way when they ask you out and you're not interested.

The best thought I have for asking a guy out is this: if you like him, take the chance. If he turns you down, it doesn't mean you're unattractive. It's no reason to give up dating. Maybe in a year or so, he will go out with you. Meanwhile, go on with life. Keep your eyes open to meeting the next someone special.

During your teens it's likely that you will turn guys down for dates, and you will also be turned down possibly many times. Does this mean you should withdraw from the human race, lock yourself in your room and forget life? Absolutely not. It means you try again. Risk, and fail; risk and win.

Paying for the date

I'm giving you my personal thoughts on this, Larissa. Who pays depends on the circumstances of the date, individual finances, and informal dating rules at your high school. You will have to decide what is best in each relationship.

For teens with an allowance or limited income, dating can be expensive. Many teens have groups of friends that go out together and each person pays her or his own way.

I think on a first date (perhaps the first few dates), the person who does the asking out should pay for the date. If you decide to keep dating, talk to each other how you both feel about handling dating expenses.

You can lead into the topic by thanking your date for the movie, dinner, or whatever you did. Tell your guy you know movies and such are expensive and you'd like to offer to pay what you can afford (50/50, 30/70). Be sure that both of you are agreeable on who pays what share.

+ Who works? He, you, both, neither?

+ Who has more "play" money?

+ Are either of you old-fashioned and feel the male should always pay? Do you need to compromise?

+ What method feels comfortable to you and your date?

When talking about money:

+ Offer only what you can afford. It's easy to feel generous and over commit yourself.

- If money problems arise, don't be afraid to talk to each other. Money misunderstandings can ruin a relationship quickly.

- Be flexible to one another's job changes or other situations which affect available income.

- Don't feel like every date has to be an expensive affair. In the winter, sledding is fun. In the summer there is the beach, the zoo, or a picnic in the park.

When girls and guys lead each other on

Males and females should always respect each other. Both sexes can feel the pain of a deception or rejection. It's not right for guys or girls to use each other. But sometime, when you want something, it's easy to forget your values just this one time.

In high school I wanted to go to a concert. I knew a guy who liked me and I knew he'd take me. I didn't like him but I wanted to see the concert. Your grandma told me that I wasn't being fair to him, but I left my conscience at home and went to the concert. He paid for everything, and of course assumed that I went with him because I liked him.

The next week he called me for another date, and I had to tell him I didn't want to date him. After that, he wouldn't look at me in the halls. I knew he was hurt, I felt like dirt. I didn't like people using me, but I had used him.

What could I have done differently? I could have paid my own way and gone to the concert with a girlfriend. I could have made it clear I only liked him as a friend and paid for half of everything. In dating you learn a lot about life. I learned a good lesson.

Boyfriends are not problem-fixers

Larissa, everyone has personal or family problems during their lives. It's easy to want someone—a friend or boyfriend—to fix the problem, take us away from it or take care of us. But a boyfriend isn't a father or big brother figure to solve problems. That type of relationship isn't healthy. Good relationships are based on independence, not dependence.

Unhealthy or Abusive Relationships

No human being deserves to be abused. If you get into a relationship with a guy who is mean to you, hits you, calls you names, or is too daring for you, get out of the relationship. If a guy is abusive, he isn't good for you. Many times it's tough to leave. You have to—for your health, safety and sanity. If you can't leave on your own, many towns have battered women's shelters that help women out of abusive relationships.

Everyone has personal problems in their lives, but we don't have the right to inflict our problems on each other. Teens raised in abusive homes may think abuse is normal behavior. The truth is abuse is wrong. It's dangerously destructive.

Any time a teen couple finds themselves arguing and fighting most of the time they're together, they need to take a good look at the relationship. Discuss what's causing the problem. Perhaps one person wants to break up, but is afraid, and masks the unhappiness in fighting and nit-picking. Or one of the partners may be jealous (with or without good reason) and that's the reason for fighting. Whatever the problem, a relationship isn't a fighting match. A relationship is caring for one another and enjoying spending time with one another.

If you get into a bad relationship, *get out immediately and don't go back.*

In school you go together and break up and go together and break up. In junior high you may not go with a guy more than one or two weeks. That's not enough time to even start a relationship. In junior high and high school all the going together and breaking up can become frustrating and make your life complicated. That's normal.

If you want to increase your chances of having good relationships and a good life, take to heart these eight points.

- Each of us counts as a human being. Each of us wants to have good friendships and relationships—and each of us can have good friendships and relationships.

- There is no life rule that says you must have a boyfriend all the time. That's like saying all girls must have green hair. Maybe you are a person who has more fun with a group of friends. What you do is right for you.

- Date only if you really like the guy. Dating to gain acceptance or status at school or to fill a void of family love or self-esteem isn't healthy for you or fair to the guy.

- If you like someone but they don't like you, it doesn't mean you're unattractive or uninteresting. It means that the two of you aren't meant to be together. There is someone else for you.

- You cannot make someone like you or love you. Yes, you can hang around that person more and make sure you're noticed, but in the end, a person will either be attracted to you or not be attracted to you.

• If you get hurt by a relationship or friendship, prolonging your hurt only puts your life on hold. You do need to mourn, so go ahead and let out your anger or tears. Then pick yourself up and get on with your life. There will be other relationships for you.

• Relationships require communication. Friendships, dating, and marriage work only when both people in the relationship communicate with each other.

• The best relationships often happen when a person isn't looking for someone. Your Uncle Tom appeared when your Aunt Cathy had had it with guys.

Except for about one percent of the teen population, teen relationships aren't forever. Your teens and early twenties are for learning about relationships so it's normal to date several different people and make mistakes.

Girl/Guy Friendships

Many girls have best friends who are guys. This can be someone you've grown up with whom you've been friends with for many years or it may be someone you met at school. He may be your age, younger, or older. You can talk to each other about anything including each other's dating dilemmas. Best friends are great. Not every girl has a guy for a best friend, but if you do that's something special. The only problem you may need to watch for is that sometimes dates become jealous of best friends. The best approach for jealousy is for you and your friend to respect the concerns of the date while assuring him that the relationship is simply a friendship. Hopefully, the date will be able to accept the friendship.

When best friends date

What if one of you suddenly develops a romantic interest in the other? Larissa, this is a tough situation and it happens quite often.

Most of the people I've talked to said their experience of dating a best friend in high school didn't turn out well. It wrecked the friendship for awhile.

On the other hand, I know of a couple who started dating after high school. The couple eventually married, and their marriage is great.

If you and your male best friend start dating and it doesn't work out, the friendship may be hurt for awhile. But if it is a strong friendship, down the road you should come back to being friends.

When best friends have sex with each other

Unless it's a case of post-high school dating, I'd say do not have sex with your best friend. This is how one teen summed it up:

> "My best friend asked me to have sex with him. I said, okay; we both wanted to see what it was like. Afterward it was terrible. Our friendship wasn't the same. He thought we should keep having sex as friends, and date other people. I couldn't handle that. We started avoiding each other. I missed being his friend. It's been a whole year and we're just now starting to talk to each other again. I hope our friendship comes back to what it was before. I never want to have sex with a best friend again—it just messes things up."

When best friends grow apart

Guy/girl friendships change just like other types of friendships. Your best friend in junior high may not be your best friend in high school. Change can hurt; but for every old friend who moves on, there are new friends to take his or her place.

Larissa, I hope I've given you some reasonable standards you can use to judge the quality of your relationships. Let me know if you have any questions about this letter and we'll work on those together.

My next letter to you is titled Going Together and Breaking Up. I think you will find it contains a lot of food for thought.

Hugs,
Mom

_____

_____

_____

_____

_____

_____

_____

_____

_____

_____

Letter 14

Going Together and Breaking Up

Dear Larissa,

Going together is nice; breaking up feels lousy. Being liked by someone you like feels wonderful; liking someone who is not interested in you hurts. But all these interactions are part of having relationships.

This letter talks about going together (going steady) and breaking up with a guy. If everyone took a course entitled Relationships in junior high, high school, and then again as adults, perhaps we'd all be better at relationships—dating relationships and friendships. I hope the following information will be helpful to you.

Going Together

Teens today said "going together" basically means the same as when I was a teen. Going together means dating only one person at a time. Once a couple has a few dates they're thought of as "going together"—until they break up.

Going together equals a relationship. Couples can have good or bad relationships. If both partners practice the qualities of a good relationship (see Letter 13), going together can be great. If one or both partners are still learning about relationships, going together can be frustrating and troublesome.

Teen dating provides you with valuable lessons in self-esteem, love, lust, jealousy and possessiveness at one of the most rocky periods of your life. Some of these lessons will be painful. Have you ever needed to bounce back from a painful experience?

The following situations are not uncommon when you are in a going together relationship.

You think your guy is cheating on you

First try to find out if the information is true. This can be tough because the information could be a rumor started by someone who wants you to break up.

If you have evidence that makes you suspect he is cheating on you, schedule some time alone together. Calmly (not accusingly) tell him you saw or heard things that lead you to think he's cheating on you. It's important to keep a cool, level head while you're talking to him. Ask him if the information true. Is he tired of going together? Does he want to break up? Wait for him to answer.

If he does not want to break up, tell him if you are going to continue going together you expect him to immediately stop whatever he's been doing.

If he wants to break up, the best thing to do is break up right there. Breaking up is tough, especially if you really like a guy. But if he's cheating on you he's not worth your time.

You break up with a guy and someone starts going with him or dating him, and then you want him back

First, be sure you are not falsely jealous. If you genuinely want him back, you may let him know it. However, it's not right to go in and break up a relationship. He may not want to get back with you. If he does, great. If he doesn't, that hurts. You may have to steer clear of him until the hurt goes away.

You like a guy who is going with someone else

Wait until they break up. It's not right to break up a relationship.

Your friend's guy and you start liking each other

This is another tough situation. One person in the triangle is going to be hurt.

+ Tell him she is your friend.

+ If he breaks up with her to date you, he'll have to wait until she gets over the break up before you and he start dating.

+ You won't date him behind her back.

This may be hard for both of you. But stop. Ask yourself how you would feel if someone were dating your boyfriend behind your back.

These are relationship situations for you to think about. Although I'm sure I missed some, the important thing to remember is that if you're faced with a situation you don't know how to handle, ask for help—from me, a friend, a school counselor.

Your job is to learn and become stronger, not to crash and burn. You can do it! Each of us as human beings possess a tough inner strength. If you call on your inner strength you can bounce back from any relationship. You can triumph over any life challenge.

Breaking Up

A popular song when I was young was "Breaking Up is Hard to Do!" Breaking up was and always will be difficult because being in a relationship means dealing with one another's feelings. Breaking up always hurts one partner or the other or both.

What if you think you want to break up? First, make sure you really want to do it. Ask yourself the following questions. Write your answers down on paper. These questions also apply to friendships.

- ◆ What first attracted you to your boyfriend?

- ◆ What things do you like or dislike about him and your relationship at the present time?

- Why do you want out of the relationship? Are you feeling smothered or wanting to date other people. Maybe there are sexual pressures or he's abusive.

- Is breaking up something you want to do or are your friends or a situation influencing you?

- Have you talked about the problem and tried, as a couple, to solve it?

If your answers indicate that you should break up, how are you going to tell him? It depends on the relationship. If your boyfriend is calm and mature, breaking up in person may be best. If he has a temper, a phone call or letter may be better so he has a chance to cool off. Here is a sample conversation. You write your own.

Steve, (or if by letter, Dear Steve)

I've been doing a lot of thinking. I can't date you anymore. I'm sorry if this is a surprise. It's what I have to do. (You may want to include the reason you're breaking up.)

If this hurts, I'm sorry. It hurts me, too. Breaking up isn't easy. There are other girls for you. It's best you find someone new. I'm sorry.

You have a feeling your boyfriend wants to break up with you

This is a tough one. You may not want to break up. But it's better to confront the possibility than hurt yourself by denying or avoiding the problem. Ask him in person, phone or write him. This is a sample script. You write your own.

John,

I've felt these last few days (weeks) that things aren't the same between us. Do you want to break up? If you do, tell me.

I'd rather not break up, but if you're not happy, we need to break up.

Wait for his answer.

If he doesn't want to break up, ask him what is bothering him. Is it a personal problem or one with the relationship? If it's a relationship problem, talk about how the two of you can solve it.

If he wants to break up, you'll want to know why. You may want to cry or scream. You deserve an answer because you are a part of the relationship, but he may not give you an answer or give you an honest answer.

Breaking up hurts. The process of getting over a relationship or friendship is similar to the process of resolving a death. There is a mourning process which can include all or some of these stages:

- Denial—"He couldn't have dumped me like that!"

- Anger—"Why that no good, so-and-so. I'll show him."

- Bargaining—"If he'd come back, I'd. . . ."

- Depression—"I can't believe it's over. What went wrong?"

- Acceptance—"Okay, it's over. We weren't right for each other. There is someone else out there for me."

Breaking up always hurts one person or the other. The hurt is real. It can feel like your whole world is falling apart. But your first breakup won't be the only one. The average female has hundreds of friendships and many relationships during her lifetime. Life is too full to let one relationship get you down. You have to heal the hurt and get on with life.

When my eighth grade boyfriend broke up with me for another girl, for weeks I was angry and depressed. I was convinced that no one loved me; I'd never have anyone else and my friends weren't really my friends. To make matters worse, my old boyfriend and his new girlfriend were around every corner I turned. My friends tried to comfort me, but I was convinced my life was ruined.

A month later a guy in band class started liking me. I found I liked him better than my first boyfriend. Now looking back on the situation, I see how I could have made things easier for myself. I shouldn't have wasted so much time moping around. My old boyfriend wasn't the only guy on the earth. A new boyfriend did come into my life.

Sometimes in break up situations, you need to avoid each other until the angry party has worked through his or her hurt.

When I broke up with my freshman boyfriend, I wanted to be friends. But when I'd say, "Hi," he'd follow me around insisting we get back together. I knew he was hurt and not thinking rationally. Even though I didn't want to, I finally had to avoid him for awhile until he cooled off. Finally he started liking someone else. The interesting development was that by our senior year, though we dated other people, we'd become close friends.

Readjustment time varies anywhere from a few days to several months to a year or more. Being obsessively depressed is dangerous; so is never grieving over your loss. When you're feeling hurt, angry or depressed, your body releases chemicals that add to that hurt, anger or depression. You can help yourself get over a break up faster by doing two things.

- Alternate your time between time to yourself and being around friends.

- Get regular daily exercise, such as walking, swimming or running. Exercise releases chemicals in your brain that counteract the chemicals that are adding to your hurt.

Keep reading. My next letter is a serious subject, about dating and sex, and should give you lots to think about.

Love you,
Mom

_____

_____

_____

_____

_____

_____

_____

_____

_____

LETTER 15

DATING AND SEX

Dear Larissa,

How far should you go sexually when you date? This is a difficult question to answer. A couple will probably hold hands, kiss, and walk around arm in arm. The closer you are to a guy romantically the more your body says, "His kisses are wonderful; I want to be physically close to him."

The stronger the physical attraction the more your bodies will want to respond to each other. However, sexual activity encompasses many different levels. Sexual involvement depends on many factors:

- Your age

- How long you and your boyfriend have been dating

- How well you know each other

- Your beliefs about sexual activity

- His beliefs about sexual activity

- Your maturity level

- His maturity level

- Whether the relationship is a good friendship, crush, lust or the beginning of a mutual like

- Your reasons for wanting to respond physically to your boyfriend; you want to show affection, caring, love, or he's cute and you're only sexually attracted to him.

There are five levels of sexual interaction.

- Kissing, hugging, holding hands

- Making out—prolonged kissing sessions

- Light petting —feeling body parts, clothed

- Heavy petting—exploring body parts under clothes or partially unclothed

- Intercourse—slang: having sex, making love, doing it, messing with—and oral-genital sex—slang: blow job, eating at the Y.

In grandma's high school days, social rules demanded that young people limit sexual activity in junior high to holding hands. Kissing, making out and petting were for high school. Intercourse was for marriage.

By my teens, we were kissing in junior high. By high school graduation about one-third to one-half of the seniors were having intercourse. Today many more high school seniors will be sexually active. Parents believe that because of sex in movies, magazines and on TV, teens are experimenting sexually at much earlier ages.

Parents are concerned because:

- Teens aren't protecting themselves against STDs. STDs, AIDS, cervical cancer, and teen pregnancy are serious threats to health, reproductivity and sexuality.

- Many teens today aren't using birth control. Teen pregnancy rates have skyrocketed.

- Young teens aren't ready to handle the emotional feelings of intercourse. They don't understand the difference between sex and love.

Respecting your sexuality and that of others is important when you date. Intercourse is the most intimate way for two people to express their love for each other. Intercourse isn't something to pass around freely like a bag of junk food. Choose your relationships carefully. Don't date people who don't respect you and who aren't kind, trustworthy and honest.

Junior High/Middle School

I believe most parents feel that junior high/middle school couples should stick to kissing, holding hands and making out.

Here are the reasons why:

- Junior high teens rarely use birth control or don't use it correctly. Girls easily become pregnant.

- Having a multitude of sex partners increases your chances of contracting AIDS, STDs, and getting cervical cancer. If you start having sex in junior high, there is a good chance you'll be a teen mom or have had an abortion before high school graduation. You've probably had several STDs. You may be HIV positive—the virus that causes AIDS. Currently there is no cure. If you don't take care of your reproductive system, you may not be able to have children later in life.

- Having sex in junior high is usually viewed as a game—have sex with someone and move on to a new partner. Sex-only dating can hurt you physically and emotionally.

High School

In high school, the question of how far should you go sexually depends on your moral convictions about sexual activity.

The heavier the making out, the greater the urge to have intercourse. Heavy petting (caressing body parts, partially clothed or unclothed) is actually the second of the four phases of intercourse. During heavy petting the man's penis becomes erect and the female's vagina becomes moist. Your body's natural, physiological response is to have intercourse. Your body tries to override your mind. It's often difficult to stop yourself from going all the way—regardless of how moral or religious you are or how frightened you may be of AIDS, pregnancy, or STDs. If you are considering heavy petting, you need to know that it can lead to having sex.

Of the many guys I dated in high school and college, there were only two with whom I could have had a lasting intimate relationship. One of those guys was your father and I married him. The other guy wasn't ready to settle down.

When the time comes that you consider intercourse, be
sure you are ready:

+ Is this something you want to do or is your boyfriend
  pressuring you to have sex? What are your beliefs
  about sexual activity?

+ Are you having sex for reasons other than a loving
  and committed relationship? Some girls and guys
  have intercourse to be accepted at school. Some people drift into sexual activity without thinking and
  then become trapped with a pregnancy, STD or
  AIDS.

+ Are you and your partner ready to handle the new
  feelings intercourse creates: love, guilt, uncomfortable-
  ness, jealousy, possessiveness, embarrassment and con-
  fusion?

+ What are the health risks? Is this the type of guy
  who's had sex with other girls before you? Unless you
  use a condom every time you have sex you're at a
  high risk for catching chlamydia, syphilis, gonorrhea,
  AIDS, or any other STD. If I was a young woman today, I would never ever have sex with a guy who
  wasn't wearing a condom.

+ What about becoming pregnant? Condoms alone are
  not 100 percent effective in preventing pregnancy.
  Are you also using a foam spermicide, the pill or
  some other form of effective contraceptive? Without
  birth control, it is possible to get pregnant anytime
  during your monthly cycle.

♦ Is this someone with whom you have a long-term relationship? Or, is this just one of many guys you'll date before marrying or settling down with one partner?

The greater the number of sexual partners you have, the greater your risk for cervical cancer and infertility from STDs.

Teens told me they have definite beliefs about sexual involvement. Some teens have religious beliefs about intercourse. They believe God intended intercourse for marriage only. Until they marry, they limit their sexual activity to kissing, hugging, holding hands, and making out.

Other teens have moral feelings about intercourse. They want heavy petting and intercourse to be with someone special—someone with whom they have a solid relationship. They know that person may not come along until sometime after high school and they are willing to wait for the right relationship.

What do you think about these beliefs?

There are also teens who think casual intercourse is fine whenever and with whomever—it's a game. Some protect themselves and their partners from pregnancy, AIDS, and STDs; others don't. How do you feel about casual sex?

Sadly, a few teens never use contraceptive or STD protection. The guys could care less if they make you pregnant or give you STDs or AIDS. The girls don't care if they spread STDs or AIDS or become pregnant. How do you feel about how these teens treat themselves and others?

Other teens have good morals, but they are in such need of parental-love or self-love that they get into sex in hopes of satisfying their love need. Unfortunately, sex alone isn't love. What do you think might help these teens?

Your sexuality is an extremely powerful force, Larissa. A touch as simple as a kiss can be arousing. But sexual involvement is intimate, mature involvement. Having sex is similar to driving, voting, and drinking. You need a certain level of maturity to handle the responsibility.

If you and your boyfriend can't talk about sexual issues—from birth control and STD protection to sexual turn ons/offs—rethink what you are going to do sexually and with whom. You have to tell each other what your sexual values are and stand by your beliefs.

How sexually active should you be when dating, Larissa? The ultimate guideline is that you should not do anything sexual that makes you feel uncomfortable, goes against your moral values or religious beliefs, or puts you at risk for pregnancy, AIDS, or a sexual disease.

In my teen years making out and petting went like this: one partner (usually the guy) would go as far as he could until the other partner (the girl) told him to stop. Teens say that is still how it works today—though the girl is sometimes the aggressor. Often because of embarrassment or fear, saying no is difficult for both sexes.

Sex on TV, in movies, and magazines gives many teens the idea that if they like each other it's required that they have sex. If they were honest with each other, many guys and girls would rather wait until they are older.

Before you begin dating or going with someone, know what your sexual boundaries are. If your guy tries to cross those boundaries, tell him you aren't comfortable going any further. Going further leads to having sex and without birth control you can become pregnant even doing it one time.

- ◆ Does he want to be a teen father?

- ◆ Do you want to get pregnant in junior high or high school? While your friends are out having fun, you will be at home feeding a baby.

It only takes one act of intercourse to become pregnant.

Two thousand teen girls per day become pregnant in the United States. Don't let this be you.

Let's take relationships a step further. Say you are in junior high, middle school or high school and are dating. You're probably playing the "Does he like me, do I like him?" game. You're learning all the rules—why we stay together and break up—and you're doing great! Then. . . one of you wants to add intercourse to the relationship. Sex changes dating and the rules of dating. In my next letter we will explore some of the differences between what guys and girls think about sex and love.

Take care of yourself,
Mom

_____

_____

_____

_____

_____

Letter 16

What Guys and Girls Think About Love and Sex

Dear Larissa,

Girls and guys view sex and love differently because males and females are different. Our bodies are different. We have different hormones. We behave differently.

Generally, boys act masculine and girls act feminine. As young children girls are more apt to reach for dolls, while boys are more apt to reach for trucks. Though males can very capably raise children, the actual nurturing instinct to have children and a home usually surfaces earlier in females.

It's important for you to understand the differences between male and female behavior because it affects dating and relationships. A good number of guys see sex in dating as a pleasurable physical activity, rather than an intimate activity of closeness. They don't see sex as like/love until they fall in love—and for many that may not be until their twenties or thirties.

On the other hand, girls are more apt to think of sex in dating in terms of like/love. In a survey of a medium-size high school, 90 percent of the guys said that when they were sexually excited, they would tell a girl anything to make out with her or have sex with her. Though many said they didn't like themselves for being dishonest, they gave in to their physical feelings.

Differences and Similarities

- Females verbalize feelings more easily and more often than males. Girls often feel they must know what the guy is thinking about the relationship—every five minutes of that relationship. On the other hand, for many a guy, if he likes you, he'll tell you he likes you and keep on liking you until he says differently. He doesn't enjoy being asked every five minutes if he still likes you. Occasionally, you can also have reverse situations in dating where the guy shares all of his feelings and the girl isn't comfortable with intimacy.

- Most people don't like to be chased—approached yes, but not chased. If a guy knows a girl is chasing him, it usually makes him run even faster to escape. It's much the same as when a guy comes on to you, too strongly, too fast.

- Often guys will say "I love you," when they mean, "I like you," and we girls immediately have thoughts of being with our boyfriends forever. Most guys aren't trying to trick girls when they say "I love you." Guys think "I love you" is what they're supposed to say.

But "I love you" can mean many things.
"I love you" can mean:

♥ I like you a whole lot (right now).

♥ I love you now when we're together but not forever. We're both in the eighth grade and forever is a long way off.

♥ I like you a whole lot (so let's keep going together and see if it turns to love.)

♥ I love you as a friend (but not as someone to date).

♥ I love you as a person (but not as a date so let's break up).

♥ I love you so I can make out or have sex with you—I'm really only using you for sex.

♥ I love you (forever); this "I love you," is the big one, usually reserved for marriage.

When you date, ask what the "I love you" you receive really means. The following summarizes some important points about love and sex.

♦ You will meet some guys who only want to date for sex (making out, petting and intercourse). These guys will say anything, especially "I love you," in order to get you to make out or have sex with them. If you get into a relationship like that, it should quickly become clear what the guy wants. If a guy only likes you for your body—not for who you are as a person—he doesn't deserve your time or friendship.

Likewise, some girls use guys to get the guys to do things for them, buy them gifts or take them places. Using people is cruel and selfish no matter who is doing it.

♦ Guys who care for you won't pressure you into anything sexual that you're not comfortable doing. And, you won't pressure a guy into anything sexual he's not comfortable with.

♦ The majority of guys do not get serious about marriage until after high school—sometimes many years after high school. Girls sometimes think about marriage while still in high school. During high school you may become serious about a guy and he is not interested. He may change his mind after high school or he may not be the right person for you.

♦ Though guys don't always show their feelings, when a guy falls for you, it can be as intense as when you fall for a guy. If you break up with a guy, it hurts him as much as it hurts you when a guy breaks up with you. Always be respectful of the other person's feelings during break ups.

Larissa, choose your friendships and dating relationships carefully. Listen to your heart, but use your brain!

With love and respect,
Mom

P.S. If puzzled by a relationship, refer back to this letter and Letters 13 and 14.

LETTER 17

MORE ABOUT LOVE AND SEX

Dear Larissa,

What is sex? What is love? It's important you understand the difference—and when sex and love interconnect.

Love

Whether platonic (non-sexual) or romantic, love is a deep caring for a person and sharing of yourself and your life with that person. You can love your friends and family (platonic love) and at the same time love someone whom you're dating (romantic love). In this letter I will concentrate on romantic love because dating is generally the first step toward romantic love.

Romantic Love

All romantic love—begins as either (1) crush (infatuation), (2) like/love or (3) lust (intense sexual attraction towards another person). People fall in love in one of these ways.

Crush (infatuation)

A crush is when you like a person, but you haven't told that person of your feelings. Usually a crush is centered on a person (a movie star, singer, teacher—a person older than you) where there is little chance that person will or can return your feelings or that the two of you will date. In seventh grade I had a terrible crush on a sophomore in high school who never even knew I existed. But I spent hours thinking about us being together. Have you had any crushes?

Like

Like is simply liking a person. You are attracted to the person's personality and looks. Like is the most stable of attractions and the one most likely to grow into love. Like is one of the foundations of a good relationship. Like is what you should strive for when dating. Have you had any "like" relationships yet?

Lust

Lust is the trickiest of attractions because lust is a purely physical and sexual attraction. A guy may have the greatest body or sexiest smile you've ever seen. You may feel you could melt in his arms. You don't know why you are obsessively attracted to this person, but your body is telling your brain that you want this guy. Never mind that once you get to know him the two of you are incompatible or he's a jerk. Lust is a giddy, energy-charged, sexual high that may happen many times throughout your life. But lust is dangerous.

Lust-only relationships don't last. Lust can easily trick you into intercourse without birth control. Lust can also trick you into a relationship where sex rather than mutual respect and caring dictates the relationship.

It's probable that during your life you will find yourself uncontrollably attracted to someone. To determine if you are in lust or like/love, take the Lust vs. Like/Love Quiz below. Check the statements that best describe your feelings about your relationship. Then use the scorecard on the next page to evaluate your feelings.

LUST VS. LIKE/LOVE QUIZ
Check Your Answers

Column 1
It's Lust

☐ Your date's "body" is the main attraction.

☐ Few qualities attract you to your date, though the ones that do may be strong.

☐ The relationship started in a matter of hours or days.

☐ Your interest in the relationship comes and goes. It's not consistent.

☐ The relationship's effect on your personality is destructive. You're moody and not yourself.

☐ You live in a one-person world. You worship your date, seeing him as faultless.

☐ Few or no friends approve of the relationship.

☐ Distance hurts the relationship— it withers or dies.

☐ Fights are frequent and severe.

☐ You speak in terms of I/me/my; he/him/his; there is little feeling of being a couple.

☐ Your ego response is mainly selfish. "What do I get out of this relationship?"

☐ You're possessive, jealous —afraid that at any minute the relationship might end.

Column 2
It's Like/Love

☐ Your date's personality and body attract you.

☐ Many or most of your date's qualities are attractive to you.

☐ The relationship develops over months or years.

☐ Your interest level in the relationship is consistent.

☐ The relationship is constructive; you're happy, calm, secure.

☐ You realistically see each other's faults, but like/love the person anyway.

☐ Most or all friends approve. You get along with each other's friends and parents.

☐ The relationship survives distance.

☐ Fights are not frequent, nor severe. Compromise for each other's feelings comes easily.

☐ You feel and think as a unit. You speak in terms of we/us/our relationship.

☐ Your ego response is unselfishness and caring for your guy.

☐ You're secure in the relationship. Possessiveness and jealousy are infrequent.

(Lust-v-Love Quiz compiled from SEX, LOVE OR INFATUATION, by Ray E. Short, copyright 1978, 1990, Augsburg Publishing House. Used by permission of Augsburg Fortress.)

Lust vs. Like/Love Scorecard

0 - 4 checked responses in Column 1
The relationship has possibilities but you need more time.
Re-evaluate monthly.

5 - 13 checked responses in Column 1
It's probably lust. The relationship might turn into
like/love but it's doubtful.

0 - 4 checked responses in Column 2
This could be the beginning of a nice relationship but you
need more time. Re-evaluate monthly.

5 - 13 checked responses in Column 2
It's likely that this is genuine like. Take your relationship
slowly. There is still much to discover about each other.

Later on in the relationship, if you think the like is turn-
ing into love, ask you guy to take this test. See if he rates a
score similar to yours.

Regarding High School Sex and Love Today, Teens Said:

"Sex is very short term."

"Love is truly enjoying being with a person whether
you're sexually active or not."

"Love is not just saying, 'I love you.' There's more to
it. You have to have feelings for someone and trust
and believe what they tell you. If a guy is with you because of sex, that's not love."

As you can see, love and sex are different. We've talked
about love; let's talk about sex.

Sex means different things depending on how the word is used. Being sexual with someone can mean activity as simple as holding hands and kissing or it can mean making-out, heavy petting, intercourse or oral-genital sex.

Having sex, (making love, doing it, messing with) means having intercourse, the man's penis inside the woman's vagina. Sharing your body like that is the most intimate way for you to be close to a guy. Emotionally, intercourse touches a deep part of your inner self. When two people give their bodies to each other they become vulnerable to each other; you lay open your soul to another person. If two people have a loving, mutual commitment, having sex is wonderful and fun. It strengthens and nurtures a relationship. But when one person is using the other person for sex or one person is more committed to the relationship than the other person, the relationship will not last. In teen dating, that happens often.

The sex drive is present in all people once they experience puberty. During puberty it's important that you begin forming personal beliefs about love and sex. Then in middle school or high school, when you have to make sexual decisions, you'll be able to stand true to your personal standards.

Having sex is emotional and physical. Physically, intercourse releases sexual tension from sexual arousal. Some people only have sex for the physical rush. For them, there is no love involved.

Other people have sex without love because they don't know how to love. Some people have been hurt by love and have stuffed their feelings. Until they risk loving again, they only experience sex on a physical level.

Still others, such as rapists, sexual abusers, and child molesters use sex for power, control or punishment. They are physically or mentally sick—and many are acting out abuse they suffered as children. They need to be stopped. They need psychological and medical help.

Intercourse between two people who care for each other can be exciting and fun. But intercourse where one person is pressuring the another person or using him or her for sex, hurts the person being used. Sex just for sex is superficial and not emotionally satisfying.

Intercourse shouldn't be added to any relationship until:

- the couple has had plenty of time to get to know each other (at least a year),

- they are mature enough to use contraceptives and STD protection,

- they are mature enough for the new emotions intercourse will bring to the relationship.

Liking or loving someone does not mean you must have sex with that person. There are many non-sexual ways for couples to be close to each other.

- Going to the movies

- Sitting and talking to each other

- Writing letters to each other

- Going dancing

- Cooking dinner for each other

- Going to the zoo together

- Feeding the ducks at the park
- Jogging or bicycling together
- Touring a museum hand in hand
- Going to sporting events, concerts or plays
- Picnicking in the park
- Riding horses
- Boating, sailing or skiing together
- Playing miniature golf, basketball or bowling together
- Skating, ice skating, skiing or sledding together
- Racing go-carts
- Doing volunteer work together

Contrary to what movies and books often portray, dating does not mean immediately having sex. However, many people today throw intercourse into relationships before they know each other well enough to be intimate.

Once you share your bodies with each other, the dynamics of the relationship change. You expect more out of each other. You or your partner may be protective, jealous, even obsessive. You or he may demand regular reassurances that the relationship is solid and going somewhere. Sometimes in teen relationships the girl can handle the intimacy but her boyfriend can't, or her boyfriend can handle the intimacy but she can't. Either way, the relationship eventually ends.

Because teen dating is generally short-term dating—weeks or months—adding sex to these relationships increases the pain when you break up. Sure you may enjoy touching and making out, but I'd like you to save the intercourse for your twenties when you have more experience with relationships and are into more long-term relationships.

Usually, guys have no idea what is pleasurable to the female during intercourse. They may have an orgasm, but they don't know how to help a girl have an orgasm. For the girl, sex is a big let-down. For the guy, he wants more sex.

One way we can release sexual tension when we are sexually excited is to masturbate. Surveys show that 90 percent of us do it. However, masturbation/self-touching is a topic that embarrasses some people. Granted, self-touching isn't something you talk about at the dinner table, but it is a perfectly healthy private activity.

Some teens think that only lesbians and gays masturbate, and that if they masturbate they're homosexual. Another common belief is that people only masturbate because they're "not getting any" (having sex). Both of these beliefs are false.

Self-touching is about being comfortable with your body. You're not gay if you touch yourself. For teen couples considering intercourse, bringing each other to orgasm through partner stimulation is a much safer way to enjoy sexual intimacy than risking pregnancy and STDs.

If you don't feel comfortable masturbating, that's okay, too. Some people don't believe in self-touching. They exercise or take cold showers. You're normal whether you do or don't masturbate.

Will you ever make mistakes dating, Larissa? Will you think a guy is fine and he turns out to be a bad date? Will you ever be lured into a situation that compromises your sexual values? It's possible.

In my junior year, during a play rehearsal a senior guy walked up to me in the curtains backstage and started pawing me. I had thought I liked him but not if he treated his girlfriends like that. In an intense whisper I told him I wasn't interested and to let me go. It was a long three minutes of intense petting that I wasn't participating in. He finally got the message. I can remember thinking as it was happening, "How do I get out of this mess?"

Everyone makes mistakes. It's whether or not we learn from them that is important. I still remember my first boyfriend, my first make out session, and the first time I felt a guy's sexual parts. Sexual expression is a normal part of growing up. Parents were teens once, too. We know all about making-out and having sex, and how confusing dating can sometimes be.

If you ever get into a sexual situation that's moving too fast for you and you're confused or scared, I'm here for you. Maybe it's a guy who comes on to you too fast. Maybe you and a guy really like each other, your making out has become intense, and you're nervous because the next step looks like intercourse. Maybe you've just had your first sexual experience, it's messing up your head and you need to talk.

I couldn't talk to Grandma about sexual issues when I was a teen because Grandma was uncomfortable talking about sex. I hope it will be different between you and me. If you don't feel comfortable talking to me, perhaps you would be comfortable talking with a teacher or another adult.

My next letter I think you'll find interesting. It deals with intercourse and how to know when it's right for you.

Here's to knowing the difference between sex and love,

Mom

_____

_____

_____

_____

_____

_____

_____

_____

_____

LETTER 18

INTERCOURSE—WHEN IS IT RIGHT FOR YOU?

Dear Larissa,

We're tackling a serious question, here. Although this letter gives you examples of why teen intercourse is not a good idea, ultimately, you are the one who makes the decision.

I personally don't believe that having sex enhances any teen or adult relationship until the couple is committed to each other for the long-term and they understand the difference between love and sex. In teen sex, there is the emotional stress of new intimacy and the reality of possible pregnancy. Current statistics show that many teens either aren't using birth control and STD protection or they aren't using it correctly or regularly.

Each day in the United States one out of every ten teenage girls become pregnant—2,000 daily!

Nine out of ten guys leave their pregnant girlfriends.

That means two out of every twenty girls and guys walking down the halls at your school will become teen parents or face abortion or adoption before they graduate. You probably know of kids in your school who are getting into sex too fast.

Because of peer pressure it's important from junior high on to be clear with yourself where you stand on the issue of teen intercourse. I personally hope you won't have sex as a young teen and that you won't ever have casual sex. I say this out of concern that your teens and twenties be free of pregnancy, STDs, and stressful relationships.

Here are comments from a couple of high school teens about having sex.

> "Wait. No matter how ready you think you are or how much you are in love, there are too many STD and pregnancy risks."

> "One night of pleasure, nine months of pain, three days in the hospital and a baby to name."

The bottom line is:

* Never have sex without birth control.

* Never let yourself be pressured into having sex.

* Don't use drinking or drugs as a source of courage to talk yourself into having sex before you're ready.

I hope as a young adult that you find a special someone with whom you can have a wonderful lifetime relationship. Just as building a good relationship takes time, being sexually comfortable with someone takes time. The majority of people do not have great first sexual experiences. Couples should be able to talk about their likes and dislikes and to feel comfortable enough with each other to be honest.

Some girls and guys' first sexual experiences are abuse situations. They are molested or raped by family members, acquaintances or friends. This is emotionally destructive and illegal. If you know anyone in that situation, have them read my letter on sexual abuse and talk to a school nurse, counselor or the local county health department immediately.

Some girls' first experiences are painful or unpleasant for other reasons. Their boyfriends force them into having sex before they are ready; the penis penetrates the vagina without the vagina being adequately lubricated. That was true in my day and teens tell me it's still true today:

"When you write this book, be sure and tell girls not to let their boyfriends pressure them. I wasn't relaxed or ready and it really hurt. I would tell younger girls to wait until they are at least eighteen and mature enough to handle it. There are a lot of emotions they will have to deal with. Most younger girls aren't ready."

"I would tell girls younger than me to wait till they're older. There are too many teens getting pregnant and having babies.

"Don't give in to peer pressure. Guys will use every line in the world to try and get you to have sex. The most common ones are, 'But, I love you' and 'I'll break up with you, if you don't.' If a guy uses either of these lines in an attempt to get sex, the girl should tell the guy to take a hike."

"Never have intercourse until you're absolutely sure you're ready, and you know you and your boyfriend really care for each other. Most guys don't really understand what love is until after high school. Make sure you know the guy's sexual history. If he's had sex with other girls, beware of STDs and AIDS. He should always wear a condom."

"Don't be fooled by fast-talking macho guys or non-talking, silent types; 99 percent of the time, they'll have sex with you and then dump you."

All the teens agreed that sex changes a relationship. If your guy really cares about you, he'll wait until you're ready and he won't hassle you. Likewise you won't hassle him until he is ready. Once you do have sex—if it is a pleasurable experience, you will probably want to continue having sex. Sexual arousal is extremely powerful. You could begin to feel like every guy you date is a candidate for sex. The truth is they're not. There will probably be only one or two guys in your lifetime with whom you could develop a lasting relationship.

Sex easily tricks people into thinking, "this guy's the one." Or, "even though this isn't exactly the guy I want if I leave him, I'll never find anyone else." I still see far too many guys and girls marrying a year or two out of high school who aren't good matches for marriage. Later they are unhappy in the marriage or get divorced. If they had looked at the relationship without the sex, they may have been able to see that it wasn't a good match.

Once you've had sex with someone your relationship will be tougher and breaking up more difficult.

If you do end up having intercourse as a teen, use birth control every time and prepare yourself for the intimacy.

Consider the following questions before adding intercourse to a relationship.

- Will the relationship become nothing but sex?

- Will sex help or hinder the relationship growth?

- What if you become pregnant?

- Do you have the money to raise a child?

- Would your guy be a caring, responsible father or would he dump you and ignore the child?

- How many of your after school plans (college, career, travel) will you have to postpone or change due to an unplanned pregnancy or early marriage?

Sex complicates relationships. If you were involved sexually with a guy, how would both of you talk to each other about these concerns?

Mom, I like the idea of waiting to have sex until I'm ready for it, but kids like to hassle people like me.

It takes guts, but if kids hassle you, ignore them and walk away. Or look them in the eye and say, "Why do you even care about my sex life? You're the one who should be worrying about AIDS and pregnancy." Larissa, you are right for standing firm in your beliefs. Choose friends who like you for you and not for your decision as to when you have sex.

Will you have sex as a teen, Larissa? If you believe that intimacy should be saved for marriage, you'll wait to have sex until you find the guy you want to spend your life with. There is nothing wrong with waiting until you're married or engaged.

I hope you will wait until your twenties when you've had some years experience with relationships. If you wait you'll be more knowledgeable about using birth control and using it correctly. You'll be able to better handle the emotional feelings of having sex. You'll also be more able to know if a guy genuinely cares about you or he's just using you for sex.

In addition to waiting until you've had some experience with relationships, there are also these reasons to consider:

- Teen Pregnancy. The objective of high school is to prepare you for living on your own. Today very few married couples can live on one income. If you want to have nice things—a home, car, clothes—you need to graduate with good grades and obtain some type of job training after high school. Becoming a pregnant teen limits your opportunities, puts your personal goals on hold, and makes life extremely difficult for you and your child.

- AIDS will kill you. Currently there is no cure. Because of AIDS you need to personally know the guy you're dating and his background. AIDS has been transmitted to the teen population. It's suspected that hundreds of teens are now carrying the virus.

♦ STDs are rampant in the teen population. Unless treated medically, they can make you infertile (unable to have children). Teens often have sex and never ask each other about their sexual histories. When you have sex with a guy without using condoms, you're having sex with everyone he has ever had sex with before. This is exactly how STDs are transmitted.

♦ The greater number of sexual partners you have in your lifetime, the greater your risk of cervical cancer from undetected STDs.

♦ When a couple jumps into sex too soon, it's easy to become so wrapped up in each other that you drop out of life, your grades fall, and you neglect your friends. Nationwide, only one-percent of high school dating relationships turn into life-long commitments.

♦ Having pre-marital intercourse would violate your moral and/or religious principles.

On the next page is a summary of dumb and good reasons for having sex. You could probably add some of your own reasons to the list.

Dumb Reasons To Have Sex	Good Reasons To Have Sex
1. Peer Pressure. So what if your friends are having sex. You control when the time is right for you. If they tease you or pressure you, they're not real friends.	1. You're married and sex with your husband is an expression of love.
2. Curiosity; to see what it's like. With pregnancy, AIDS, and other STD health risks, this is not safe.	2. You're in a long-term committed relationship. You want to share your love with each other, and...
3. One-night stand. You meet a guy at a party. You like him, but you don't know him. With AIDS and STDs, casual sex is out. Don't risk it.	a. You're not going against your moral or religious beliefs.
4. You think it will make you grown-up. You grow up; sex immediately complicates your life.	b. You know each other to be free of AIDS and STDs.
5. You're pressured into sex by a boyfriend. You think by doing it, you will keep or catch him. This plan usually backfires.	c. You feel that you are both mature enough to handle the intimacy of sex. You've talked to each other about having sex. You know that adding intimacy to your relationship will affect your relationship in new ways.
6. You let drinking or drugs be your excuse.	
7. You do it to be popular. This backfires and gives you a reputation.	
8. You do it to defy your parents or get their attention.	d. You reach a mutual agreement to have intercourse.
9. Confusing sex for love. You want to be loved so you substitute sex for love.	e. You've decided on and purchased the type of birth control you'll use.

You're Not Yet Ready For Sex

If you feel you are not ready for sex, there are some things you can do to minimize your chances of getting into sex.

* Respect Yourself. Don't use sex in hopes of keeping or catching a guy. If your guy pressures you about sex, tell him you care for him, but you're not ready. If he truly cares about you, he'll wait. If your guy doesn't stop pressuring you, break off the relationship.

* Limit your time alone with your boyfriend, if you are not ready to have sex and don't have much will power in passionate moments.

* Don't drink or use drugs. Alcohol and drugs distort your thinking. You can easily get into sex without birth control and STD protection if you drink or take drugs.

You are a sexual person. Your hormones can be so active you may feel like your insides are bouncing off the walls. Your sexuality is a real part of you. Relationships are a part of growing up. But having sex before you and your partner are mature enough to handle the intimacy only causes hurt.

At what age will you have intercourse? It's different for everyone. When you become sexually active depends on your moral beliefs and values. You should not have intercourse until you're mature enough and ready to properly use birth control and STD protection every time.

When you have intercourse is your decision. If you feel that religiously or morally sex should be saved for marriage, then wait until you're married or engaged. If you have sex as a teen, you need to be responsible about birth control, and prepare yourself emotionally for the new feelings sex will bring to your relationships.

After reading this letter, you'll know that the decisions you make about sex will affect your life in many ways. I know you care about yourself. I know you'll be responsible.

Choose well. Be sure before you jump.

Mom

_____

_____

_____

_____

_____

_____

_____

_____

_____

LETTER 19

SEXUAL DISEASES

Dear Larissa,

Sexually transmitted diseases (STDs) and AIDS are nothing to mess around with. STDs can make you sterile (unable to have children). AIDS will kill you and currently there is no cure. In 1992 the fastest growing number of HIV-positive cases—the virus that causes AIDS—was among teens. In your school, one out of three sexually active teens will contract an STD each year. This could be you or one of your friends.

Here is one high school senior's story:

> "Since my junior summer I've had sex with two guys, both of them I was going with. I knew the guys weren't virgins, but I never thought I'd catch an STD. I figured our crowd was safe. When I went for my pap smear, the doctor said I had chlamydia. I was embarrassed. If my doctor hadn't discovered

it, over time it could have made me sterile. Some day I want to have kids. Now I think twice before I add sex to relationships. If I do have sex, the guy always wears a condom."

Some STDs are passed between a couple through intercourse, but a number of STDs can also be transmitted through heavy petting and oral-genital sex. Obviously, the surest way to avoid STDs is to be abstinent. If this is not what you choose, you will have to protect yourself against STDs and AIDS in all your sexual relationships.

Warning signs that a person may have an STD are:

- Unusual discharge from the vagina or penis.

- Itching, burning, sores, rashes or redness on vulva or penis.

- Pain or tenderness in the genital area or lower abdomen.

- Pain or burning feeling when urinating; frequent urination.

If you ever have any symptoms, see a doctor immediately.

Protecting Your Body From STDs

Buy and keep condoms in your purse

Always use condoms, never let down your guard —"Oh just this one time won't matter." Don't wait until you are in a passionate embrace. Be prepared. Never have sex with any person you suspect isn't practicing safe sex.

Condoms should never be reused.

Condoms can be bought at any discount store, pharmacy, or convenience store. County health departments usually have free or inexpensive condoms. If you're embarrassed, go with a friend and purchase them together.

Talk frankly with your sexual partner about STD protection before you have sex

"Brandon, I like you and this relationship. If we are going to have sex, I insist on a condom every time. Condoms are for both our protection. *No Condom, No Sex.*" You control the situation. Be ready and able to help your partner put on the condom.

Use only latex condoms with spermicide for each act of intercourse

Let's be honest about this; some guys don't like condoms and will refuse to wear them. If this is the case, you must be tough. *No Condom, No Sex.* Until doctors come up with a miracle vaccine for STDs, unprotected sex is not safe.

Look before you love

Any sore, rash or discharge your partner has may be a symptom of an STD. If you suspect anything, do not have sex. Do not engage in any heavy petting. Do not engage in oral-genital sex.

Postpone having sex until you're ready and then, be choosy about sexual partners

Although condoms are the best protection (other than abstinence), they are not 100% effective. Our sex drive is very powerful. Once you have sex, it's easy to add sex to every relationship. People who wait until their twenties to add sex to relationships are more apt to use STD protection properly and regularly.

Have a pap smear and vaginal examination every year.
Ask to be tested for any STDs prevalent in your area.

If you find a marriage or life partner, before marrying
each of you should be tested for AIDS and be
checked for STDs.

Below are listed the ten most common Sexual Transmitted
Diseases (STDs) affecting both males and females. There
are other less well known but equally dangerous STDs.

Ten Most Common STDs— Affecting Both Males And Females

AIDS (HIV virus)
Increasing among heterosexuals, especially teens.
Spread through oral-genital sex or anal or vaginal intercourse.
Symptoms: No early symptoms; later swollen glands, fever, diarrhea, night sweats, weight loss and fatigue.
Treatment: No cure. Early testing recommended, medications help retard onset of full AIDS.
Damage: Eventually death.

CHANCROID
More common in warm climates than cold.
Spread by skin to skin contact.
Symptoms: Herpes-like sores, or ragged-edged pimples, or bright red blisters, on genitals or elsewhere on body.
Treatment: Antibiotics.
Damage: Open sores on genitals make it easy to pick up the HIV virus and other STDs.

CHLAMYDIA (NGU in men)
Fastest spreading STD in U.S. among fifteen to twenty-five year olds.
Spread through intercourse and close sexual contact.
Symptoms: Called the "silent" STD, because there may be no initial symptoms until infection has began to damage reproductive system.
Later painful urination, discharge in men; pelvic pain, itching, discharge, bleeding between periods in women.
Treatment: Antibiotics.
Damage: Causes sterility, ectopic pregnancies (outside the uterus usually in the fallopian tubes).

GENITAL WARTS (HPV, Human Papilloma Virus)
750,000 new cases a year, teens very susceptible.
Spread through intercourse or oral sex.
Symptoms: One to three months after contact, very tiny flat, or cauliflower-like bumps appear inside/outside genitals.

Ten Most Common STDs (Continued)

Treatment: Warts frozen off or burned off with laser or electric needle.

Damage: Risk of genital cancer.

GONORRHEA (clap dose, drip)
1-2 million cases a year, mostly people under twenty-five-years-old.
Spread through intercourse, heavy petting if genitals touch.

Symptoms: frequent painful urination, discharge—sometimes no symptoms.

Treatment: antibiotics.

Damage: Sterility, arthritis.

HEPATITIS (Type B)
Very Common. Type B which is sexually-transmitted is the most dangerous.
Spread by sexual contact, uncleanliness.

Symptoms: Dark urine, yellow eyes, tenderness in liver area, also flu like symptoms.

Treatment: Bed rest. Weeks, months to recover.

Prevention: Hepatitis vaccine, as a child or adult, usually available at county health department.

HERPES SIMPLEX VIRUS-II
(genital herpes)
500,000 to one million new cases each year.
Highly contagious, spread by sexual contact, genitals and mouth.

Symptoms: Painful blister-like sores on genitals.

Treatment: Acyclovir eases pain, shortens attacks, but there is no cure.

Damage: Once contracted virus lives in body forever, and sores reoccur when person under stress. Sores painful, can cause blindness in babies of mothers who have active herpes. Uninfected sex partners are always at risk.

Note: Cold sores—herpes simplex-I is not genital herpes-simplex-II.

PUBIC LICE (crabs) and SCABIES
Common in crowded living spaces.
Highly contagious, spread mostly by sexual contact, close physical contact, contaminated towels, toilet seats, bedding, clothing.

Symptoms: Lice live in pubic hair; mites (scabies) burrow under skin. Severe itching, reddish zigzag furrows under skin.

Treatment: Creams, lotions and shampoo. Keep clean, bathe/shower daily.

Damage: Lice can carry other diseases.

SYPHILIS (Syph, Pox, Bad Blood)
Infection rate at highest level in forty years.
Spread by direct contact, usually sexual intercourse.

Symptoms: Painless red sores on genitals. Sores disappear, but disease remains in body to reoccur again.

Treatment: Penicillin or other antibiotics.

Damage: If not treated, syphilis can cause paralysis, dementia and death. Sores make it easier to contract AIDS.

TRICHOMONIASIS (Trich)
Caused by tiny parasites that live in moist places in body. Common STD, but prompt treatment cures.
Spread by sexual contact, shared damp wash clothes and towels, shared swimming suits.

Symptoms: Discharge with bad odor, frequent, painful urination.

Treatment: Best treatment is prevention. Wear cotton underwear, use condoms and spermicidal foam.

Larissa, we only receive one body. It has to last us our entire lives—from our teens on.

Protect your body at all costs. Don't let STDs get control.

With love,
Mom

_____

_____

_____

_____

_____

_____

_____

_____

_____

Letter 20

Birth Control

Dear Larissa,

In Letter 18, I discussed what you should consider before deciding to have sex. I also told you that I hope you're in your twenties and in a committed relationship before you have sex. Whether a teen has decided to have sex or not, she or he should be familiar with the various types of birth control and the importance of using contraceptives—every time, no exceptions, anything less is like playing Russian roulette.

That is what this letter is about. I'll give you some general information about contraceptives and then discuss in detail each of the available contraceptives and effectiveness rates.

This information is so important because of the crisis of un-wed teen mothers and rampant STDs. There is a lot to cover. Let's get started.

Once the decision has been made to have sex, both partners should be involved in the process of learning about contraceptives. You and your partner should go to a family planning class and learn about the different contraceptives available. Then use contraceptives every time you have sex.

If your partner won't go to the birth control class with you, ask yourself if he is as committed to the relationship as he says. Contraceptives are the responsibility of both partners.

How do I get contraceptives?

I will make an appointment for you with our family doctor if you feel comfortable with that. If not, there are other alternatives. You can find them listed in the phone book or ask your friends.

Clinics take after school appointments—some have evening and Saturday hours. The health clinic accepts all ages, and your visit is strictly confidential. If no clinic is available in our town, you may have to drive to a neighboring town or county for services.

Some contraceptives, such as the pill, Norplant®, Depo-Provera®, and the diaphragm will require a visit to a doctor or clinic.

What if I'm not sure that a clinic assures confidentiality?

When you call for an appointment, ask the clinic if they ensure confidentiality. Be sure to get the name of the person you talked to. If they say yes, by law your visit is confidential.

Can I buy non-prescription birth control at a pharmacy or convenience store without going to a clinic?

Yes, you can buy non-prescription contraceptives such as condoms, foams, and sponges, but they are only effective against pregnancy when you use them correctly. At some schools, you can go the school nurse to get the information you need. The family planning class can help you and your partner learn how to correctly use these forms of birth control.

How do I get to the clinic if I can't drive?

Ask your partner or a girlfriend to take you, or you can ask me. In the city, you can take the bus.

Should my boyfriend go to the clinic also?

Yes! Birth control is the responsibility of both the man and the woman. Boyfriends need to know what kinds of birth control are available, how your body works and why it's essential that females have yearly pelvic examinations.

Today many couples visit family planning clinics together. Even if your boyfriend is older and has been to a clinic before, he should go with you for your moral support and to learn any new information that is available.

Don't put it off. If you even think you might have sex, obtain birth control before the first time you have sex. If your boyfriend won't go to the clinic with you, you may want to question his commitment to the relationship.

What will happen when I go to a family planning clinic, county health clinic, or our family doctor?

Usually a nurse or receptionist will greet you at a check-in desk and ask you to fill out a form asking for your name, birth date, health status, and other important information.

If it's your first visit, you and your boyfriend will attend an initial information class on family planning covering information on contraceptives, STDs, and necessary body care such as annual pap smears and monthly breast exams.

Afterward, you will be taken for a weight, urine and blood check. Then you will be taken to a private examining room for your breast and pelvic exam, pap smear, and doctor consultation. Exams are necessary to make sure you are free from sexual diseases and cancer.

In the examining room a nurse will ask you to remove all your clothing and cover yourself with a paper or cloth sheet. When the doctor arrives she or he will give you a breast and pelvic examination, take a pap smear and talk with you about the type of contraceptive you want to use. Following the examination, you can usually pick up your contraceptives at the cashier's window before you leave.

Usually at health clinics if a male doctor examines you, a female nurse will be in the room. If this is not so and you are uncomfortable, ask that a female nurse come in so the examination can continue.

How much will the exam and birth control cost?

Contraceptive costs vary depending on the type. At county and Planned Parenthood clinics, fees are based on your income. At most county and Planned Parenthood clinics, birth control is available to you free of charge if you don't have a job, allowance or other income. Purchasing supplies month by month can ease the expense by spreading the cost out over time.

What does a breast, pelvic exam, and pap smear involve?

Almost every young woman is concerned about her first breast and pelvic exam and pap smear—I was. Now my yearly exam is routine. I even prefer it over six month dental check-ups.

If you are mature enough to have sex, you are mature enough to have an annual exam. When you start having sex you need an annual exam for prompt detection and treatment of STDs and cervical cancer. Young women who aren't sexually active, usually don't need annual exams until they reach age eighteen.

When I went for my first exam I was nervous. I didn't have a book to read to tell me what to expect. I calmed myself by talking to myself:

"I am a mature person. I care about my body. Having an exam is part of keeping myself healthy. I will breathe deeply and relax. I'm having an exam because I care about my body."

Calming myself and deep breathing helped me relax. Soon my annual exams were easy. If you're nervous when it comes time for your first exam, you might try talking to yourself. Soon your annual exams should become a simple routine.

The Examination

The examination itself is normally broken into three parts: breast exam, pelvic exam, and pap smear.

Breast Exam

The breast exam consists of the doctor palpating (pressing) your breast with her or his hands to detect any abnormal lumps or cysts. You should also perform this procedure monthly on yourself right after your period. Many clinics have plastic examination reminder cards you can place in your shower or near your tub as a monthly reminder. Ask the doctor if these are available.

Breast cancer currently affects five to ten percent of all females. You are at greater risk if there is a history of breast cancer in your family. Since early detection substantially increases the rate of recovery, monthly breast self exams and yearly mammograms after age thirty-five should be a priority for all women.

Pelvic Exam

To ready you for the pelvic exam and pap smear, the doctor will ask you to slide your buttocks to the edge of the examining table, place your feet in stirrup supports, and open your knees.

If you are squeamish, now is the time to breathe deeply and concentrate on your weekend plans or run multiplication tables in your head.

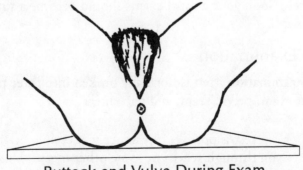

Buttock and Vulva During Exam

The doctor will put on a pair of thin, sterile, latex gloves and sit at the end of the table. She or he will likely turn on a bright lamp aimed at your genital area. The warmth from the lamp is soothing and should help you relax. During this time the doctor can usually take cell samples for any STD testing you request.

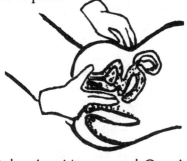

Palpating Uterus and Ovaries

Most doctors will first palpate your uterus and ovaries for any signs of abnormalities such as cysts or tumors. The doctor generally does this by inserting two fingers into your vaginal canal while her or his other hand presses on your groin area just above your pubic hair. You will feel a little pressure, but the exam only lasts a few seconds.

Pap Smear

The pap smear consists of the doctor taking a speculum (a small, metal or plastic appliance) and inserting it into your vagina to slightly open it. The doctor then inserts a soft cotton swab into your vagina and gently scrapes sample cells off the cervix. These cells are sent to a lab for detection of cervical cancer. If you relax, this procedure is not uncomfortable; you'll hardly feel anything.

Usually, if you don't hear from your doctor, the test is negative. If your test is positive, the office will confidentially contact you through school or some other means. Having a positive test does not mean you have cervical cancer; occasionally tests will turn up false positive. It does mean you will have to take a second test.

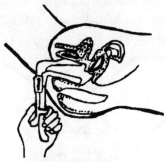

Pap Smear—Speculum In Vagina

After completing the three exams, the doctor should discuss which contraceptive is best for you. Then the doctor will excuse her or himself to allow you to get dressed. If you're at a health clinic you can usually pick up your birth control before you leave. If you're at our family clinic, the doctor will write a prescription which you'll fill at a pharmacy.

Ask the doctor or nurse questions during any part of your exam or the information session. No question about your health is a dumb question. Reproductive care is vital to your health. You need correct information.

What if I'm really squeamish about having a pelvic exam?

Be honest. Tell the nurse and doctor so they can help you relax. Breathe deeply and think of anything other than the exam. If you want additional support, request that you have someone (me, a girlfriend, your guy) with you during the exam.

How often do I need to go to the clinic?

Generally, exams and a pap smear are performed once a year.

* * *

Larissa, the following information gives you contraceptive effectiveness rates and details the various methods. Before you become sexually active, read and reread this information carefully.

The three most effective (greatest success of preventing pregnancy) forms of birth control currently available for females are Depo-Provera® (the shot), Norplant® (the five-year contraceptive implant), and oral contraceptives (the pill). Although nothing "synthetic" is natural for your body, contraceptives were developed to be as compatible with your body as possible.

The pill, shot and implant do not protect you from STDs.

The pill, shot or implant should not be used if you think you might be pregnant, have, or have had blood clots or vein inflammation, high blood pressure, migraines, liver disease, unexplained vaginal bleeding, an abnormal growth, or cancer of the breast or uterus. Also, if you have a family history of diabetes or other generational diseases, your doctor may run tests to see if you can use these contraceptives.

Sexual intercourse without birth control results in pregnancy

BIRTH CONTROL CHART
In order of effectiveness re: typical use

Abstinence (not having intercourse)—100% effective. Of 100 girls, zero will become pregnant.

Sterilization (surgical vasectomy—males, tubal ligation—females)—100% effective. A permanent birth control method for persons who have decided they absolutely do not desire any more children.

Norplant®, (five-year contraceptive implant). Studies show effectiveness greater than the pill; 100 girl comparison not available.

Depo-Provera®, (the three-month shot). Studies show effectiveness greater than the pill; 100 girl comparison not available.

The pill (oral contraceptive)—97% effective. Of 100 girls, three may become pregnant during first year of use. Women who take the pill at the same time daily, have less than a one percent chance of becoming pregnant.

Male condom—88% effective—more effective with foam. Of 100 girls, twelve may become pregnant during first year of use.

Female condom -two types now available. 100 girl comparison not available.

Sponge—82% effective for females who have not had a child. Of 100 girls, eighteen may become pregnant during first year of use. For women who have had a child, twenty-eight may become pregnant.

Diaphragm/Cervical Cap with Spermicidal Jelly—82% effective. Of 100 girls, eighteen may become pregnant during first year of use. High ineffectiveness rating may reflect incorrect usage.

VCF, Vaginal Contraceptive Film—effectiveness comparable to that of other spermicides—foams, jellies, suppositories, 100 girl comparison not available.

Suppositories/Foam/Jellies—79% effective. Of 100 girls, twenty-one may become pregnant during first year of use.

IUD —a prescription contraceptive that only women who have had a child and who are in a monogamous relationship may use. Of 100 women three may become pregnant during first year of use.

Fertility Awareness Method W/Abstinence—76% effective. Of 100 girls, twenty-four may become pregnant during first year of use. This is an involved and somewhat complicated method of charting ovulation, this birth control method is not recommended for young, unmarried women.

Information compiled in part from: J. Trussell, R.A. Hatcher, W. Cates, F.H. Stewart, and K. Kost, "Contraceptive Failures in the United States: an Update," *Studies in Family Planning* 21 (1), 1990.)

Non-contraceptives—these are not effective

Douche—0% effective. Not a birth control method. Douching will not kill sperm. In fact some researchers believe that the washing action actually propels the sperm into the cervix.

Withdrawal—0% effective. Not a birth control method. Guys always say, "I can withdraw before ejaculating." That doesn't matter. Pre-ejaculatory semen from the penis empties into the vagina before ejaculation. It doesn't matter if a guy withdraws before he ejaculates because sperm from the pre-ejaculatory semen is already in your vagina, swimming upward to find an ovum.

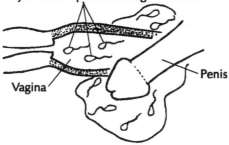

Pre-ejaculation sperm heading for uterus

Vagina

Penis

Withdrawal—0% Effective

Drugs—0% effective

Marijuana, crack, cocaine, acid; using drugs does not affect male sperm development or a woman's ovulation cycle to the point that it prevents conception. A person high on drugs usually forgets all about birth control and STD protection.

Abortion—abortion is not a contraceptive. Abortion is a medical procedure to terminate a pregnancy.

Contraceptive Facts

Only abstinence and condoms will protect against STDs. All other forms of contraceptives are used for birth control only.

Abstinence (not having sex)—100% effective, birth control and STDs

Abstinence (not doing it, not going all the way) is the only 100% effective way of not becoming pregnant. Kissing, hugging, caressing, and holding hands are ways to show your love for each other without having sex. If couples engage in petting or orgasm by partner stimulation, extreme care must be taken that semen does not get anywhere near the girl's vagina. Sperm close enough to the vaginal opening can find their way into the vagina.

Advantages: No chance of pregnancy. Relationship is easier and less complicated. You don't have to hassle with the stress intercourse puts on a relationship.

Read instructions and follow the your doctor's advice before using contraceptives.

Possible Problems: Couples who have gone together for a long time and are into heavy making out have to use strong will power to avoid the temptation of having intercourse.

Norplant®—99% effective

The Norplant® implant is a five-year low dose contraceptive consisting of six small, soft, flexible capsules placed under the skin of the upper arm. Norplant® works by continuously releasing levonorgestrel which inhibits ovulation. The implant usually can't be seen unless the woman is very thin or muscular. Once they are in place, the capsules will not move around or break. If a woman desires pregnancy, the implant can be removed before the five-year time limit.

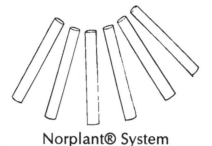

Norplant® System

Advantages: Reliable pregnancy prevention for a five-year period. Convenient, no hassles, constant protection.

Possible Problems: High initial cost, though very cost effective for five-year period. Must be implanted by a health care provider. Placement and removal may leave small scar. In some women, side effects may be greater than if taking the pill. Side effects can include prolonged menstrual bleeding, unexpected bleeding, nervousness, enlargement of ovaries and/or fallopian tubes, acne, excessive growth of body hair, or hair loss.

Depo-Provera® (the shot)—has been used in some countries for more than thirty years.

Depo-Provera® (drug name: serile medroxyprogesterone acetate suspension, DMPA) is a contraceptive shot that is administered by a health care provider every three months (you get shots four times a year). Depo-Provera® works by stopping your body from producing menstrual blood, so a fertil-

Depo-Provera®

ized ovum has no blood rich uterus lining to attach to.

Advantages: Effectiveness rating greater than the pill. Constant three month protection. Cost spread out over a year in quarterly payments as opposed to the high initial cost of an implant.

Possible Problems: You must remember to get your shot on time, or you will not be protected against pregnancy. Some people don't like shots. Side effects may include: bloating, weight gain, headaches, depression, lost of interest in sex, hair loss.

The Pill (oral contraceptive)—97% effective

The Pill is still the most popular form of birth control for young women because:

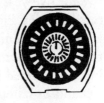

* the majority of females can take the Pill,

* it's easy and convenient to use,

* it's initially less expensive than an implant.

Oral contraceptives work by changing the level of hormones (progesterone, estrogen) in your body so you don't ovulate (produce a fertile egg) or build up the endometrium (lining of the uterus) in your uterus. By preventing these activities, no conception (pregnancy) occurs.

Pills come in a variety of hormonal types, levels, and monthly cycles. When taken correctly the pill is 97 percent effective in preventing pregnancy. Oral contraceptives are safe for many women and may have fewer side effects than the implant or shot. You and the doctor can determine if you can take the pill and which pill will suit you best. In certain cases the pill has had medical value in reducing severe menstrual disorders: excessive menstrual bleeding, severe cramping, iron-deficiencies, pelvic inflammatory disease, non-cancerous breast tumors, ovarian cysts, and ovarian and endometrial cancer.

Pill Facts To Know

* To be effective the Pill must be taken the same time each day. Many people get pregnant by not taking their pill at a set time each day (example 7 a.m. daily or 5 p.m. daily) If you forget a pill, call your clinic immediately for further instructions. Never "borrow" a pill from a friend. It could be the wrong dosage, and it breaks her cycle of pills. If you even skip one pill, you could easily become pregnant.

* Antibiotics and certain cough medicines affect the Pill's effectiveness. Use a second form of birth control to prevent pregnancy.

* When starting the Pill you must go through one month's pill prescription before the Pill will protect you from conception.

* Oral contraceptives are safe for many women, though you might experience mild side effects. If any of these symptoms become severe, call your clinic immediately.

* Medical opinions vary on how many years a young woman can take the pill. Many doctors contend that the Pill can be used until your early thirties, then you should switch to another type of birth control. Other doctors advise taking Pill breaks. You are instructed to take a break and go off the Pill for a few months

once every few years. If you have sex during this time, be sure to use another contraceptive. Also, do not start and stop pills every other month between boyfriends. Constant stopping and starting oral contraceptives is hard on your body and may decrease the pill's effectiveness.

Advantages: When taken correctly, it is an effective contraceptive with few side effects for most women.

Possible Problems: Some women experience side effects, such as bloating, slight weight gain, headaches, depression, and mood swings. You must remember to take the pill daily.

Condom—88% effective for birth control; 98% effective against STDs

The condom (rubber, prophylactic) is a sheath of strong, thin latex (rubber) that a male rolls onto his erect penis before intercourse. If the condom does not have a premolded reservoir at the end to contain the semen after ejaculation, the male must leave slack in the end of the condom to hold the semen. Some condoms are made with reservoirs, others are not. Condoms are so thin, neither male or female should sense any loss of feeling when using them.

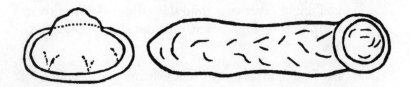

Rolled-up and Unrolled Condom

After intercourse, the male needs to hold on to the condom to prevent it from slipping off his penis while he pulls his penis out of the female's vagina. He should then carefully remove the condom from his penis and throw the condom in the trash. A new condom must be used for each act of intercourse.

Condoms are inexpensive, reliable, and easy to buy as a primary or secondary birth control method. They are available in a variety of colors and styles and can be bought without a prescription at almost any pharmacy, grocery store, or convenience store. Girls can carry them in their purses, guys can carry them in their wallets.

Caution: When carrying condoms in your purse or wallet, throw out your supply every two months and purchase a new supply. Over time the latex can crack, making them unsafe as birth control and STD protection.

Do not use Vaseline® or petroleum jelly as a vaginal lubricant with a condom. The Vaseline® and jelly can dissolve the rubber.

Young couples should not be embarrassed to use condoms. Couples can put the condom on the penis together, as foreplay before intercourse. To be most effective in preventing pregnancy, condoms should be used with contraceptive foam. The male wears the condom; the female inserts foam into her vagina.

Advantages: Non-prescription, easy-to-buy, and inexpensive. Condoms are currently the most effective form of protection against STDs.

Possible Problems: Semen can leak from the condom if the penis is not withdrawn properly from the vagina or rough handling of the condom tears the latex.

Female Condoms

Two types of "female" condoms are available. Made of thin latex, they cover the inside of the vagina. These condoms are fairly new as a form of birth control. When the time comes that you need birth control, ask a doctor about the female condom's usage and effectiveness rating.

Sponge—82% effective for women who have not had a child

The vaginal contraceptive sponge is a soft, bell-shaped synthetic sponge approximately two inches in diameter filled with a chemical to kill sperm. A nylon loop is attached to the bottom of the sponge to aid in removing the sponge.

The sponge works by blocking the entrance to the uterus (cervix) and releasing a spermicide that kills the sperm.

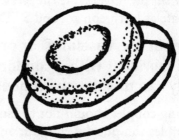

Sponge Contraceptive

Because of the chance of toxic shock syndrome never reuse a sponge, never use a sponge during menstruation and never leave a sponge inserted for more than twenty-four hours.

To be effective, sponges must be left in at least six hours after intercourse. Then they should be thrown in the trash.

Advantages: You don't need a prescription to buy the sponge; one size fits all. Insertion is easy. The sponge can be inserted in private, hours before having sex. Intercourse can be repeated once within a twenty-four hour period.

Possible Problems: Removal problems can occur. If you can't remove the sponge, call the health clinic immediately for removal. Some people may have an allergic reaction (burning, itching) to the spermicide and can't use the sponge. There is also some concern that sponge users may be at an increased risk of toxic shock syndrome (TSS) (also associated with tampon use).

Warning Signs of TSS: Fever, chills, vomiting, itching, irritation of the genitals, persistent unpleasant odor or unusual discharge from the vagina—visit a doctor or clinic immediately.

Diaphragm With Cream/Jelly—82% effective

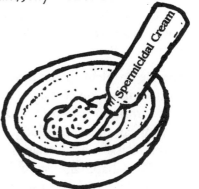

The diaphragm is a soft rubber disk with a flexible rim that is used with contraceptive cream or jelly. The diaphragm comes in different sizes. It is a prescription contraceptive and must be fitted by a doctor. To use the diaphragm, fill it with contraceptive cream and insert it into your vagina before intercourse so that it covers

Diaphragm With
Spermicidal Cream

your cervix. Once in place, the diaphragm can't be felt by either you or your partner. It stops the sperm from entering your cervix; the cream or jelly kills the sperm.

To be effective, your diaphragm must be left in your vagina six to eight hours after your last intercourse before removing it.

Diaphragms last anywhere from one to two years before needing replacement. Always check your diaphragm frequently for tears or pin holes by holding it up to the light.

The diaphragm is a good choice for women who can't take the pill and women whose partners object to condoms. However, the diaphragm usually isn't prescribed for young unmarried women unless they are comfortable touching their bodies and are responsible about using birth control every time. Using a diaphragm means a commitment to using birth control every time.

Advantages: Once learned, insertion is easy and you and your partner can't feel the diaphragm. Many women feel that the diaphragm is not as messy as the sponge or condom. There are no side affects like those which can occur from the Pill.

Possible Problems: Even though most women have no side effects, some women may experience mild allergic reactions to the cream or jelly used with the diaphragm. The diaphragm can become dislodged during sex if the woman is on top or if she has a relaxed vagina as a result of childbirth. The diaphragm should be refitted after each childbirth or if you gain or lose more than fifteen to twenty pounds. If there are pregnancy symptoms, genital itching or irritation, frequent bladder infections, unusual vaginal discharge, and discomfort when the diaphragm is in place it should be reported to your doctor immediately.

VCF (Vaginal Contraceptive Film)—used in Europe for eighteen years

Vaginal film is a thin, clear square of material containing a spermicide. The female puts the film over her middle finger and inserts her finger into her vagina so the film is placed on her cervix. Insertion takes practice; it's recommended that the woman practice inserting a few films before using one for intercourse. Her fingers must be completely dry before touching the film.

The film must be inserted not less than fifteen minutes and not more than one hour before intercourse. Once in the vagina the film dissolves into a thick gel that coats the cervical opening, killing sperm on contact. The body's natural fluids wash the gel away. A new gel must be used for each act of intercourse.

Advantages: Easy to use, few if any side effects and can be bought without a prescription.

Possible Problems: Must be used correctly to prevent pregnancy, not 100 percent effective. Not available in all stores at this time.

Suppositories/Foams/Creams/Jellies—79% effective

These products are chemical substances inserted deep into the vagina before intercourse to kill the sperm while not harming vaginal tissue. Suppositories, foams, creams and jellies are available in a variety of dosages and names. If not used exactly as directed, these products may not form a good barrier to the uterus and pregnancy can result.

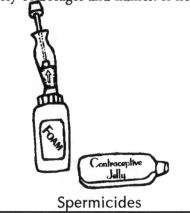

Also, most brands are only effective at killing sperm one hour after insertion. To increase effectiveness these products should be used with a condom.

Spermicides

Advantages: These products can be bought by anyone at any age and they are fairly easy to use.

Possible Problems: Some women may experience genital irritation. Switching brands may help relieve the inflammation. Others may have an allergic reaction to any spermicide and can't use this form of contraception. Some women complain of leakage and messiness.

Rhythm Method (fertility awareness with abstinence)— 76% effective

Fertility Awareness or "Rhythm Method" or "Natural Family Planning" is a natural form of birth control that uses your body temperature and vaginal mucus to chart your ovulation cycle. Once you determine the most fertile times during your cycle, do not have intercourse during those times. This method is not recommended for teens because of its low effectiveness rate.

Advantages: The rhythm method is natural; you aren't putting any kind of contraceptive in your body.

Possible Problems: Its low success rate means pregnancy is more probable. It requires continual tracking of the menstrual cycle.

Sterilization—100% effective

Today, sterilization (vasectomy for men, tubal ligation for women) is an increasingly popular form of permanent birth control for parents who have their families and don't desire more children or for couples or individuals who don't want to be parents.

Now that you've read about the different types of contraception, which ones do you like?

Larissa, having sex is a matter of personal values and deciding when you can handle the responsibility of using birth control. When you need it, this chapter will be here for you to reread. I know you'll take care of yourself and when the time comes you'll use birth control and STD protection.

I love you,
Mom

_____

_____

_____

_____

_____

_____

_____

_____

_____

Letter 21

Teen Pregnancy

Dear Larissa,

Of all the letters in this book, this letter I wish I didn't have to write. I hate the fact that so many girls become pregnant. Life is full of obstacles. Teen pregnancy creates many additional obstacles for the girl, the baby and the father of the baby. But when girls are asked why they didn't use birth control, the number one answer is; "I didn't think it would happen to me."

U.S.A. Today Magazine (January 1994) reported that recent studies suggest, "There is a common perception in this country that teenage pregnancy is somehow a problem of minority groups, but white teenagers account for 68 percent of all adolescent births in the U.S. and over half the births to unmarried mothers." Minority Americans make up the remaining teen pregnancy numbers.

In the same article U.S. A. Today Magazine reported:

- Of all American female teenagers having premarital sex, most are not consistent contraceptive users.

- As a result, an estimated 40 percent become pregnant at least once before age twenty, and four-fifths of these pregnancies are unintended.

- Twenty percent of teenagers bear a child. These rates of pregnancy and childbirth are the highest among Western industrialized nations.

- In families headed by fifteen to twenty-one year-old females, more than four-fifths of children are poor. . . .

If you have sex without birth control you will become pregnant; if not the first time probably within the first six months.

Tragedies of Teen Pregnancy

I hope you can tell from what you have read that pregnancy and childbirth are a serious commitment not to mention the approximately eighteen-year commitment to the new human being. This is a commitment you, as a teen, should never have to deal with. There is too much to learn, see and do in high school to be tied down with a pregnancy and then a baby to raise. But some girls today as young as twelve and fourteen, think they want to get pregnant to have a baby for someone to love them. A baby is not a way to get love. Being a teen mom is a twenty-four-hour baby-sitting job that never goes away. You lose your friends, your fun, your freedom, your life.

Substituting sex for parental love

Most parents sincerely love their children, as I love you. I try to show you that through words and actions—supporting your school interests, feeding, clothing, and housing you and yes, worrying about you. "I love you; be careful." "Drive carefully, the roads are slick tonight."

But when parents become bogged down in their own problems—work, home, personal issues—sometimes they don't give their children the attention needed. Other parents, although they love their children, don't know how to show love. That's not good, but it happens.

When you don't get parental love, it's natural to seek love and attention from someone else, and for girls that's often a boyfriend. A boyfriend holds your hand and kisses you. You feel loved. It's easy for these feelings to lead to intercourse, without using birth control. Then you get pregnant and you're really in a mess. No matter how much a person wants it to work, sex doesn't replace parental love or self-love. Sex for love only makes you feel more empty inside.

If there are times you need someone to listen to you, but I'm running around absorbed in my own thoughts, sit me down and say, "Mom, remember me? I need a hug." Or, "Mom, I have a problem and I need to talk to someone about it." We all mask our feelings sometimes. I don't necessarily know you're having a problem, unless you talk to me.

If you have a friend whose parents aren't available for her and she needs an adult tell her to seek out a family friend, relative, or teacher. I'll also be happy to listen to her if she feels comfortable with that.

I know when you make the decision to have sex you will use birth control. I also know that sometimes contraceptives fail. I pray you never face a teen pregnancy.

What Would Happen If as a Teen You Did Become Pregnant?

The first thing I hope you'd do is tell me. A pregnancy, planned or unplanned, is a dramatic event in any female's life. Choosing what to do with an unplanned pregnancy is a big decision to make by yourself. I love you. I don't want to see you hurt. I hope you don't make any decision before thinking about how that decision would affect your life now and in years to come.

Would I be shocked when you first told me? Probably. I might ask: "Are you sure you're pregnant? Were you using birth control? Does your boyfriend know you're pregnant?" Please realize that these are a parent's normal first reactions because pregnancy, especially teen pregnancy is a serious matter.

What would happen next? If you hadn't taken a home pregnancy test, I would have you take one. If the test is positive, we'd sit down and talk about your options. If your boyfriend acknowledges the pregnancy, you should consider his feelings about the pregnancy. However in many states according to law the female makes the final decision because she carries the pregnancy in her body.

If a young woman decides to carry her pregnancy to term she needs prenatal care immediately and then continuing care throughout the pregnancy.

Option 1: Have the baby and give it up for adoption

If you aren't ready to become a mother and you don't believe in abortion, putting your baby up for adoption is a good option. Adoption agencies have waiting lists of caring couples who can't have children of their own and desperately want children. These couples are screened as to their ability to love and nurture a child and give him or her a good home. Some states have open adoption laws where you can actually select the couple who will adopt your child, and receive reports from them as to your child's development.

Option 2: Have the baby and keep it

After carrying the baby inside for nine months and giving birth to the child, some teens feel they can't give their babies up for adoption. Raising a child is a serious responsibility. If you became pregnant today, would you be ready to accept the responsibilities of teen motherhood?

Becoming a mom means putting your child's needs first. It means missing many school activities and times with your friends. It means finding and paying for a responsible baby sitter for your child when you want to be with your friends. Will the father of the child help you financially? Is he able to be a good parent? If the father won't be involved, are you prepared to be a single mother?

Being a single mother means continuing with school to earn your diploma and working to pay for food and clothes for your child. It's almost impossible without a high school diploma to get training for any type of good paying job and without a good paying job you can't support yourself and a child. Diapers, formula and child care are expensive.

Some young mothers receive welfare; but there is no guarantee welfare will always be available.

Many teens work hard to be good moms and good providers, but it's a tough life. For teens who can't handle the stress and responsibilities, grandparents often end up raising the kids. In abuse or neglect cases, a teen's children may be taken by child custody services.

If you and the father love each other, you may decide to have the baby, finish school, and get married. I knew a couple who did that and they are still a happy family today, but they are unique.

Nationwide, less than one-percent of teens who create a child together end up marrying; 99 percent of guys still dump the girls they get pregnant.

Option 3: Abortion—terminating the pregnancy

Larissa, aborting a pregnancy is also an option that some girls choose. The girls may feel that they are not ready to be good mothers or they could not handle the pregnancy.

Abortion is a touchy subject in America. People are divided by their moral and religious beliefs about abortion. To form your beliefs you need to know both pro-abortion and anti-abortion thinking.

Some people have strong religious beliefs about abortion. They believe that "humanness" is present at the moment of conception when the sperm fertilizes the ovum. Therefore abortion at any stage of pregnancy is murder—killing human life.

Other people don't believe that humanness begins at conception, so early abortions are permissible. They believe that later in the pregnancy when the embryo grows into a fetus and displays human features that "humanness" is present.

Still others believe that a pregnancy is a growing life. They would not choose abortion for themselves, but they believe abortion is a private decision for each woman.

A few people don't view a pregnancy as a growing life. They think abortion is fine, anytime.

Whose is correct? I know that for myself and my friends abortion is a deeply personal issue. The idea of terminating a pregnancy raises many questions.

- Should abortion be permissible in rape and incest cases?

- Is it right for a rape or incest victim to have to carry the pregnancy?

- In medical situations where the pregnancy is endangering the mother's life, should the pregnancy be aborted to save the mother's life?

For many years, abortion was illegal in all states. In 1973, the Supreme Court ruled that abortion was legal. In 1990, the decision of keeping abortion legal was given back to each individual state.

Laws are constantly changing. When you read this, abortion may or may not be legal in our state. If abortion is not legal in one state, it may be possible to obtain a legal abortion in a neighboring state. Medically speaking, abortion is a safe medical procedure only when performed by a licensed doctor under sterile conditions. If performed before the twelfth week of pregnancy, abortion is actually physically less harmful to the female than carrying a pregnancy to term. However, for young women with strong family/religious ties, abortion can be emotionally disturbing.

Legal abortion costs range from $200 for an early-term abortion to over $2,000 for a late-term abortion. If someone chooses to abort a pregnancy, it is best to do it in the early stages (first three months of the pregnancy).

If you believe that abortion at any stage of pregnancy is murder, than the safest way to prevent an unplanned pregnancy is to not have sex until marriage—or if you do have sex, always use birth control. What are your feelings about abortion?

Mom, I appreciate knowing you would support me should I ever become pregnant before marriage, but I have some friends who are afraid to talk to their parents. Other friends of mine could never tell their parents. is there anything they can do?

Good question, Larissa. If one of your girlfriends becomes pregnant, if at all possible, she should tell her parents. Telling parents you're pregnant is a tough thing to do. Their reactions may be shock, hurt, and/or anger. But most parents really love their children and will want to help a daughter in this situation.

If a girlfriend feels she absolutely can't tell her parents, have her call the local family planning clinic or county health clinic immediately. These clinics have professional, caring nurses and counselors who will help your girlfriend consider her pregnancy options. The important thing is to not put off calling someone for help.

Larissa, as a teen I was never faced with a teen pregnancy. I'm thankful I never had to make a decision to be an unmarried mother, give a baby up for adoption, or terminate a pregnancy.

The bottom line is that if you use birth control responsibly, you probably won't have to worry about an unplanned pregnancy. And if you make the choice to not add intercourse to high school relationships, you will not have to worry about teen pregnancy.

Take care of yourself, Larissa. Be responsible with your sexuality. I'm always here if you want to talk.

Mom

_____

_____

_____

_____

_____

_____

_____

_____

_____

LETTER 22

SEXUAL ABUSE

Dear Larissa,

No one should ever force you to participate in any sexual activity—including intercourse—or touch you sexually without your consent. Your body is yours. No human has sexual rights over another human.

This letter is about sexual abuse, incest, child molestation, and rape. If you are ever a victim, tell me immediately. If for some reason you feel you can't tell me, tell the principal or counselor at your school or call our local county health clinic. If the first person you tell doesn't believe you, keep talking until someone does believe you.

Sexual abuse is a crime, Larissa. It's a crime because one human is violating the body of another human. Sexual abuse causes psychological injury to its victims. Serious bodily injury including the transmission of STDs and AIDS also occur frequently.

Sexual abuse is not new. Its destructiveness dates as far back as pre-biblical days. The difference is that today victims can get help; then they could not.

People sexually abuse and rape other people for many reasons. For most abusers, sexual abuse is a way to exert power or control over someone. The abuse isn't for sexual satisfaction. Other abusers are repeating the sexual, mental, or physical abuse they suffered as a child. Others are mentally ill.

Sexual abuse can range from a one-time incident of someone pressing themselves against you sexually or touching your breasts to a parent's repeated intercourse with her or his child. Sexual abuse can also be verbal abuse where the abuser manipulates the victim verbally, without physical touch. Sexual abuse is widespread. It's estimated that one out of three girls and one out of six boys will be sexually abused in some manner before their eighteenth birthday.

Larissa, it is important that you know the types of sexual abuse, the effects of sexual abuse, and ways you can lessen your chances of being sexually abused. Sexual abuse happens in high school relationships, yet it often goes unreported. Both boys and girls are sexually abused. For you, this letter will focus on female sexual abuse.

Incest

Incest is defined as any sexual activity between members of an immediate family or step-family, other than normal wife/husband sexual relations. Incest most often occurs between father and daughter or between older brother and younger sister.

Incest is serious. It's the type of sexual abuse most often kept secret or denied. Current statistics show that incest oc-

33333333

curs in one out of every four families. The victims are usually threatened by their abuser or they feel ashamed so they never seek help.

Incest causes victims to have very confused feelings about love, sex, and self-worth. Unless treated, these feelings can haunt victims throughout their adult lives affecting their relationships with a spouse, family, friends, and society.

Larissa, I had a friend in college whose older brother had intercourse with her beginning at age twelve. My friend told her mom, but her mother didn't do anything. The mother had also been abused by her brothers when she was a teen and because she had not had counseling she was not capable of responding to her daughter's need.

Note: Brothers and sisters age five and under may "play doctor" or "mommy and daddy." This type of sex play between young children is fairly common and normally is not incest. Being forced to have sex or play sex games with an older brother or sister is incest.

I have another friend who told her mother her father was forcing her to have intercourse with him. Her mother refused to believe her because the reality of what the father was doing was too painful for the mother to face. She was afraid that if she confronted her husband, she'd lose him.

Today, both of these women's personal lives suffer from those experiences.

Child Molestation

When I was eleven, Larissa, we went to a cousin's wedding dance. An old, distant uncle of mine asked your Grandma if he could dance with me. He kept pressing closer and closer to me on the dance floor and I could feel his penis becoming hard. He was a lonely widower, but trying to feel sexual with his eleven-year-old niece was wrong. When the dance ended, I told Grandma I didn't want to dance with him anymore, and I didn't.

Another friend of mine, as a child was baby-sat by her Uncle. He repeatedly molested her—touching her genitals, sticking his finger into her vagina and forcing her to touch his penis. She never told her mom because she was scared her mom wouldn't believe her. She never received any counseling to help her come to terms with the abuse. Today memories of that abuse still bother her and affect her life negatively.

Child molestation is the same as incest, but the abuser is not an immediate family member. However, the abuser may be a relative—Cousin Jim, Grandpa Bill, Uncle George. The abuser may also be a family friend or business person—Neighbor Bob, Dentist John, Doctor Carl or a complete stranger. Though this type of abuse is called "child" molestation, the law covers any victim under age eighteen. Molestation may include touching of the genitals or breasts, and having oral-genital sex or vaginal or anal intercourse.

Incest and child molestation are crimes. Perpetrators (abusers) should not be allowed to continue these activities. When the victim (child or teen) reports an abuse the abuser should get punished and/or treatment and the victim get the counseling she or he needs.

Rape

Rape, in any form, is defined as a person forcing sexual intercourse (vaginal or anal) on another person against her or his will. In the United States a woman is raped every six minutes. The majority of rape victims are between the ages of fifteen and nineteen.

Acquaintance/Date Rape

In 60 percent of rapes, the rapist is someone the victim knows—the victim knows her abuser or she is dating him. Many acquaintance/date rapes go unreported. The victim feels in some way the rape is her fault. She shouldn't have been with that person in the first place. She was drinking or doing something else she wasn't supposed to be doing. Humiliated and fearing punishment from parents, teen victims often never tell anyone about the rape. But victims should talk. A victim who can't confide in her family should tell a school counselor or the local county health clinic.

If you should ever be raped or sexually abused in any way, I want to know about it. Any type of rape and even attempted rape is traumatic. It's important that you talk to a therapist, so you can resolve the trauma and go on with life. It's also important for your health that you have an STD and pregnancy check.

Even if you were doing something I cautioned you against or if you were in the wrong place at the wrong time, I won't punish you. The abuse itself is devastating. I know. I was raped.

It was at college. I was raped by a guy a friend of mine was dating. I was at my friend's apartment for a birthday party. Early in the evening I flirted with my friend's date. I was trying to forget about the break-up with my boyfriend the night before so attention from another guy was nice.

Later that night when I went to get my coat from the bedroom, my friend's date followed me, closed and locked the door and pinned me down on the bed. He put his hand over my mouth and started unzipping my jeans. I froze when I realized what he wanted. I had always thought I could fend off a rape—no problem—but I was too shocked, and ashamed, to move. After he left, I got up, went home, curled up in my bed and cried.

The next day I told my friend what had happened. She could hardly believe her guy had raped me. She made me go to the school counseling clinic and visit with a counselor. She told the guy their relationship was over. The counselor helped me calm down. She also scheduled me for another visit to help me work through my feelings and rebuild self-esteem. Later, I was able to put the rape behind me.

At the time I didn't report the rape to the police. I thought that somehow, someway, I should have been able to stop it. In reality, the rape was not my fault. Had I known then what I know now, I would have pressed charges. Who knows how many more girls this guy might rape.

Whether it's a chance meeting, a first date, or a long-term relationship, acquaintance/date rape can happen to any woman including you, Larissa. In the United States one in every three girls is sexually assaulted in some way by age eighteen. But all too often female victims are so shaken by the abuse they won't seek help or press charges. They think, "I must have done something wrong." "I'm too embarrassed to ask for help." "I can't risk asking for help. If my abuser finds out he will hurt me (or leave me)." Sexual assault is never the victim's fault, even if she was in the wrong place at the wrong time. Rape is a crime. If you are ever raped or sexually abused, seek help immediately.

To learn how to protect yourself from rape and sexual abuse, practice these safe-guards. It's also good to take a course on self-defense.

Protecting Yourself Against Incest, Sexual Abuse, and Rape

- Stay away from people you don't trust and those you feel uncomfortable being around. If someone repeatedly engages you in sexual talk, repeatedly touches you, or brushes her or his body up against yours, tell me, a teacher, school counselor, or social worker. We want to help you deal with the person.

- If confronted by an exhibitionist (flasher), keep your cool. Don't say anything. Turn away and walk to the nearest phone, dial 911 and report the incident. Flashers are normally harmless, but don't take chances. Never provoke one.

- If someone—a relative, friend, acquaintance, or stranger tries to abuse you sexually, there are three steps to follow: (a) Say "No!" (b) Get away. (c) Tell someone what happened—me, a teacher, your school counselor, the police.

- If you are currently being sexually abused, don't protect the abuser any longer. Report the abuse. Talk to me, a teacher, your school counselor, or the police immediately.

- Don't drive around alone with a guy you don't know or you've just met—especially older guys. Even harmless looking guys can be trouble. Our world is a violent place. Young women are kidnapped and raped every day.

◆ Never take a ride home from school or work with a guy you don't know, a guy you've just met or any suspicious person.

◆ Follow your intuition. If something feels wrong, it probably is. Get out of the situation immediately. Mean what you say, and say what you mean. No is *no*!

◆ If you ever find yourself under attack, a hard blow by your knee or fist to the attacker's penis and scrotum can render him helpless for a few seconds so you can escape. A hard hit by both palms of the hands to the attacker's ears is another option.

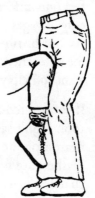

◆ If you begin liking a guy whom you don't know well, ask friends and classmates about him. If you hear that a guy is trouble, he probably is.

◆ Some guys will incorrectly take a girl's dress, body language, gestures and sexual comments as invitations to have intercourse. It's normal to flirt when you like a guy, but use common sense.

- When you leave school, a school activity, a dance, or party with a new date, let a responsible friend know what time you're leaving and where you're going.

- Do not leave school, a school activity, dance, or party with someone you don't know or someone you've just met.

- Don't make out with a guy you've just met.

- Don't get in a situation where you are alone with a guy who has been drinking or taking drugs. You may tell a guy who has been drinking or taking drugs no sex but once he has an erection, he may not take no for an answer.

You and your friends can probably think of additional ways to guard against rape and other forms of sexual abuse.

Incest, molestation and rape are frightening experiences. They leave you with confused feelings about yourself, sex, love, and relationships. There are people who can help. If you have been or know of someone who is being sexually abused. Call your local county health clinic, local sexual abuse hot-line, or the national child abuse hot-line (800-422-4453). Professional mental health counselors are trained to help you rid yourself of the bad feelings and feel good again. It's important after any type of sexual abuse to talk with a counselor to help you resolve the trauma of your incident.

If you should ever be raped or abused, come to me or the police immediately. Do not shower, change clothes, or wipe down any part of your body. Obtaining a conviction on a rape is difficult unless the prosecutor has adequate hair, clothes fiber and semen samples. Any of the perpetrator's hair, clothes fibers, and semen found on your body are evidence. I or the police will see that you're taken to a clinic or hospital where trained nurses will take hair, cloth, and semen samples from you, and then let you shower.

Larissa, while you were growing up, I tried to be alert to any sexual abuse. As a child I told you that no one (family member or anyone else) should ever touch the private parts of your body or play sex games with you. To our knowledge no one has. If I missed an incident, tell me or someone who can help. Get help now.

Larissa, this letter is not intended to frighten you, but to make you aware that sexual abuse is, unfortunately, a part of our society.

Most of the relationships in your life will be good, but should you ever encounter sexual abuse, reread this letter and get help.

All my love,
Mom

_____

_____

_____

_____

_____

_____

_____

LETTER 23

MARRIAGE

Dear Larissa,

I can't talk to you about sex and love without a letter on marriage. You may be saying, "Mom, I'm just learning about guys, I don't want to hear about marriage!"

Don't misunderstand me, Larissa. I'm not pushing you to get married. If a couple is serious in high school, I think both partners should graduate and live on their own before marrying. Your life goals usually change significantly between age eighteen and twenty-five. But sometimes you date a guy during high school (perhaps you fall in love) and you begin thinking, "What if we were married. . .?"

High School Marriages

In high school your dating can become serious, in part because your sexual feelings are intense. A few sixteen, seventeen and eighteen year-olds do fall in love, get married, and have good marriages. Be careful. What you take for love could be sexual lust. Sex alone won't keep a marriage together. Of high school marriages, one out of every two end in divorce before five years of marriage.

High school marriages fall apart because people change after high school. Your goals change. Your outlook on life changes. Life is much different after graduation, than it is living at home your junior and senior years of high school. You may swear you and your boyfriend won't change, but you do.

In a marriage when one partner grows and matures and the other doesn't, if either person can't adjust to the change, a split develops in the relationship that can lead to divorce.

But in high school when you think you're in love, it's easy to become so wrapped up in your guy that you want to marry immediately. The statistics are that the majority of men and women do not find their marriage partner in high school. Nationwide only one percent of high school seniors find their life partner in high school.

Larissa, during high school if you and a guy become serious about marriage, please consider getting separate apartments after graduation. Date for a year before setting a wedding date. If your feelings for each other are real, they will grow stronger during that year.

I saw many of my friends marry right after high school. Within five years they divorced. The same thing happens today. People marry too early and for the wrong reasons.

How do you know if both of you are in love and he is the right guy?

Unfortunately, the love that leads to marriage is hard to describe, Larissa. When it happens, you'll feel that this particular dating relationship is different. If you're both in love and thinking of marriage, you should both have a contented, peaceful feeling. But this feeling rarely happens on the first few dates; it builds as your relationship builds and grows.

How do you know when you're both ready for marriage?

That's the tricky part. Throughout your life, you may fall in love more than once. But the guy you fall in love with may not be in love with you, or he may be in love but not ready to marry.

There are two guys I thought of marrying before I met your Dad. One wasn't in love with me; the other wasn't ready for marriage. It wouldn't have worked to marry either of them.

You'll both know you're ready to marry if, despite normal engagement jitters, you feel comfortable with the decision. It's better to cancel the wedding than to go into a marriage with only one of you committed to it.

If you fall in love in high school, don't rush into marriage. Graduate, move out of the house and date for a while. Have a long engagement to be sure that you are right for each other.

Approximately one in 100 people find a husband or wife in high school. The majority of people don't marry until their twenties or thirties.

Before you marry make sure that "you" or "your guy" isn't. . .

- Marrying to get out of the house, or to quit school.

- Marrying for a father or mother figure to take care of you.

- Marrying for someone to love you.

- Marrying because it's the thing to do.

- Marrying thinking you'll learn to love your spouse later.

- Marrying because it's great sex. Sex is only a small part of marriage and it won't keep a marriage together. But sex can easily trick you into thinking this guy's the one!

Too many people marry for the wrong reasons or marry before they are ready. These marriages usually end in divorce. Do you know people who rushed into marriage and it didn't work?

Marriage Checklist

Check which statements apply to your relationship. Statements not checked should be talked about with your guy and a compromise reached before you walk down the aisle.

- You both compromise to meet each other's needs and wants.

- You're at ease talking to each other. You're not putting on a false front for one another.

- You know each other's work, career and personal goals. You're committed to supporting each other's goals.

- You both realize that marriage is a partnership and requires support from both partners for the rest of your lives.

- You know each other's views on religion, sex, money, marriage roles, male/female careers, economic status, family, and child-rearing. You've talked through the compromises that are needed.

- You both enjoy some of the same interests, but you don't have to do everything together.

- You both know that a marriage needs affection to last. You're both comfortable expressing your affection—hugs, kisses, cuddles, and I love yous. You aren't afraid to ask each other for a touch or big hug after a tough day.

- You both want to be married.

The Realities of Marriage

Marriage is work. A marriage takes both partners to make it work. But when you love someone the work isn't difficult and the rewards are great. However, marriage isn't without arguments, disagreements, trials, and pressures. Like the traditional vows: marriage is for better for worse, through good times and bad, through sickness and health.

During my marriage to your father, we've had a lot of money and no money; we've both been sick at times; we've both gone through job changes and age changes that were good and bad. But facing the good and bad together is what makes a forty year marriage as strong, loving, and exciting as a first year marriage.

Don't marry thinking that once you are married you will change your guy. The number one mistake people make is thinking they can change their partner once they're married.

People can't change other people. A guy who is immature, selfish, demanding, rude or lazy before marriage will be that way after marriage unless he changes himself. Do you want to put up with bad habits for the rest of your life?

It is possible to love someone who would not make a good marriage partner.

Mom, how are my friends with divorced parents supposed to have good role models for marriage?

Good question, Larissa. Many teens today have divorced parents. But they can learn about marriage from their divorced parents by sitting down and talking to them. "Why did you and Dad (or you and Mom) marry? Why did you divorce? If you could redo the experience, what would you do differently?" They can also read books on what makes marriage work, why people divorce, and how to know when a couple is ready for marriage. Just because teens have divorced parents doesn't mean that those teens, as adults, can't have good marriages.

Divorce

Most people don't plan to divorce. But it happens and divorce hurts. It breaks up families and is hard on children. If people didn't rush into marriage so quickly, if they took the commitment of marriage seriously and they worked at their marriages once they were married, the divorce rate wouldn't be so high.

Before You Marry

Before you marry be sure you and your guy are both in love and committed to being married. Fall in love with your heart and your head.

During your engagement talk, talk, talk to each other. Usually couples are so taken by love, they never discuss each other's views on the real issues of marriage—job goals, household chores, money, children, personal goals—until after the wedding ceremony. They say "I do," then find out later that their views about marriage are worlds apart.

Share with each other your expectations of what marriage will be like. Tell each other your future career, money, family, housing, and leisure goals. Do you know he wants to buy a speed boat? Does he know your dream is to travel? Is he a spender while you're a saver? Do you want a professional career, while he enjoys manual labor?

Understand fully each other's dreams, likes and dislikes before you walk down the aisle. While your goals may change over the years, your marriage will have a better chance of success because you started with shared expectations.

When You Marry

Once married, these housekeeping activities can help keep your marriage strong, happy and healthy.

- Talk with each other—daily. Don't let disagreements and disappointments fester. Practice forgiveness. No marriage is perfect, because people aren't perfect.

- Learn to laugh at yourself. Maintain a sense of humor about life and marriage.

- Commit to keeping your marriage alive and growing. Review that commitment to yourself morning and night.

- Nurture your love. Kiss each other good morning and good night. Hug. Cuddle. There is nothing better than a spouse's warm, loving, hold-me-tight hug after a bad day.

♦ Regularly make time among work, family, and friends to date each other and spend quality time together.

♦ Before going to sleep each night, hold each other and thank each other for the chores each of you do that become boring but keep the marriage moving—making dinner, washing clothes, repairing the car, parenting the children.

♦ Create a budget for yourselves. Include (1) a savings account, (2) a separate emergency savings, and (3) a weekly personal allowance for each of you. Work out the kinks in your new budget; then adjust that budget according to job and career changes.

♦ If serious problems arise over money, sex, careers, religion, children, or in-laws, see a professional marriage counselor or mediator to help solve the problem and put your marriage back on track. There is no shame in seeing a counselor. Couples should work with marriage counselors at the first sign of trouble instead of waiting until the trouble has progressed to the point of divorce.

Marriage is compromise—an agreement to live your lives together, caring for and loving each other.

Marriage isn't. . .a fairy-tale romance, a parent figure to take care of you, or you as the parent figure taking care of someone.

Good marriage partners are best friends, spouses, and lovers. You want to grow old together. You're a team, a pair, a couple.

I hope as an adult that you find someone you want to share your life with, and I wish you only the best.

All my love,
Mom

_____

_____

_____

_____

_____

_____

_____

_____

_____

_____

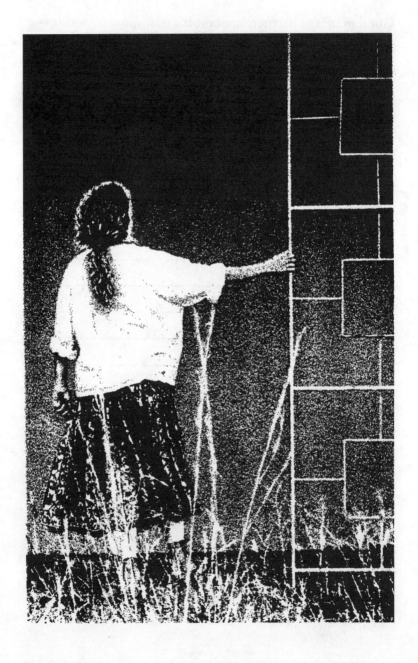

Letter 24

I Love You, Goodnight

Dear Larissa,

This is my last letter in this collection. I hope I've given you information you can use to become comfortable with your sexuality, keep healthy and make responsible dating decisions. If there are a few thoughts I would have you carry with you always, they are:

- Don't be afraid to be your own person. Love yourself for who you are. Stand firm in your beliefs and values; remember that other people are entitled to their beliefs.

- Above everything else, finish high school. Then after high school obtain some type of on-the-job training, technical schooling or college so you have a job skill to support yourself.

- Protect your sexuality. Sexuality isn't something you pass around to everyone as if it were junk food to be eaten and you, the wrapper, thrown away.

- Take care of your body. If you do have intercourse before you marry, use birth control every time to protect yourself against pregnancy. Use condoms to protect yourself against STDs.

- Enjoy your teen years. If you date, great. If you don't date, that's fine, too. Some people don't become interested in dating until after high school; they have a group of friends with whom they do things together.

- Whenever you need to talk about anything—guys, sex, love, friendships, life—I am here for you. I will try to be a good listener, open-minded and not judgmental. I'm also here if you just need a hug after a bad day.

Larissa, you're a beautiful young woman. I wish you nothing but happiness. Even though we argue sometimes, as all moms and daughters do, I will always love you and I'm proud to be your mom.

All my love,
Mom

_____

_____

_____

_____

_____

Glossary of Terms

ABORTION. Termination of a pregnancy. There are two types of abortions; spontaneous abortion (miscarriage) and induced abortion. Spontaneous abortion occurs when the body naturally aborts the pregnancy because it cannot sustain the pregnancy. It usually happens before the twenty-fifth week of pregnancy. Induced abortion is a surgical procedure done by a licensed doctor when a woman chooses to terminate a pregnancy, or when a pregnancy is endangering a woman's life and must be terminated.

ABSTINENCE. Not having intercourse, the only 100 percent effective method of not becoming pregnant or contracting many STDs.

ADOLESCENCE. The time period—normally between eleven and nineteen years—of a person's mental maturing toward adulthood.

AFTERBIRTH. See placenta.

AIDS (Acquired Immune Deficiency Syndrome). STD. A deadly disease caused by a virus that attacks the body's immune system. AIDS is spread by contaminated body fluids and blood, usually through some type of intercourse or sharing unclean needles used to inject illegal drugs. Currently there is no known cure for AIDS. (See also page 154.)

AMNIOCENTESIS. A test usually given to high-risk pregnant women (those over thirty-years-old, or women who were taking drugs or had an illness upon conception) to determine if the baby may have birth defects. The test is done by inserting a needle through the woman's belly into the baby's placenta and extracting a sample of amniotic fluid which is then checked microscopically.

ANAL INTERCOURSE. The insertion of the penis into the anus. A high-risk activity for AIDS and other sexual diseases.

ARTIFICIAL INSEMINATION. Method of impregnation of a woman by insertion of sperm inside her vagina through a small tube. Artificial insemination is an option when regular intercourse does not result in pregnancy.

BIRTH CONTROL. Avoiding pregnancy by using contraceptive protection during each act of intercourse.

BIRTH DEFECTS. Medical problems that babies are born with such as under-developed limbs or internal organs, blindness and other problems. Birth defects can be caused by a variety of reasons: defects in the ovum or sperm, inherited problems from either parent, the mother being exposed to harmful drugs or radiation during her pregnancy, and the mother's body being too young to properly nourish the baby (teens having babies), premature births, and lack of oxygen to the baby during birth.

BISEXUAL (slang AC/DC). A person who engages in both heterosexual and homosexual relations.

BREASTS. Human mammary glands. The female breasts produce milk for the baby after childbirth. The male breast does not develop to accommodate milk production. Breasts are a source of sexual pleasure for most women and some men.

CERVIX. Opening to the uterus located at the top of the vagina.

CAESAREAN SECTION. Surgical operation of cutting through a mother's abdomen and the wall of her uterus to deliver a baby when vaginal delivery is not an option.

CHANCROID. STD. (See page 154.)

CHILDBIRTH. The process in which a baby is pushed out of the woman's uterus and vaginal canal when it is ready to be born.

CHILD MOLESTER. Person who inappropriately fondles children and teens, and/or has sexual relations with them.

CHLAMYDIA. STD. (See page 154.)

CHROMOSOMES. Portions of the ovum and sperm that contain genetic information including hair color, bone structure, skin color, eye color, and sex.

CIRCUMCISION. A surgical procedure dating back to biblical days removes the loose flap or foreskin covering the end of the male penis. Circumcision is usually performed within twenty-four hours of a healthy birth.

CLIMAX. See Orgasm.

CLITORIS (slang: clit). A small, nerve sensitive pleasure organ located in the soft folds of skin just above the females urinary and vaginal openings. Stimulating the clitoris through masturbation, oral sex, or intercourse is the way most women achieve orgasm.

COITUS. Another name for sexual intercourse.

CONCEPTION. The uniting of ovum and sperm. Fertilization of an egg by a sperm.

CONDOMS (rubbers, prophylactics). Contraceptive device of thin latex rubber that fits on the penis and holds the semen during intercourse.

CONTRACEPTION. The prevention of pregnancy. Various methods used include condoms, the pill, the contraceptive sponge.

CONTRACEPTIVE SPONGE. Form of birth control. A sponge that works by blocking the entrance to the uterus and releasing a spermicide.

CUNNILINGUS. The male orally stimulates the female's external sex organs.

DIAPHRAGM. Form of birth control. The diaphragm is a soft rubber disk with a flexible rim that is used with contraceptive cream or jelly. It is inserted into the vagina so that it covers the cervix. It is a prescription contraceptive and must be fitted by a doctor.

DOUCHE. A naturally or commercially prepared solution of filtered water and other ingredients that rinses and cleanses the vagina. Not recommended, unless under doctor's orders because douching can harm the vagina's natural acidity balance.

EJACULATION. When an erect penis releases semen and sperm through intercourse, masturbation, or wet dreams.

EMBRYO. A human organism from forty-eight hours after conception to the end of the eighth week of development.

ERECTION (slang: hard-on, boner). Temporary hardening or stiffening of the penis caused by increased blood flow to the spongy tissue inside the penis. Generally, erections are caused by sexual thoughts or stimulation, but spontaneous erections happen for no particular reason.

ESTROGEN. Hormone produced by the female ovary gland. Maintains female secondary sex characteristics.

EXHIBITIONIST. A person who exposes her or his sexual organs in public.

FALLOPIAN TUBES. Small slender tubes about the size of spaghetti that connect a female's ovaries to her uterus.

FELLATIO. The female orally stimulates the male's penis.

FETUS. Unborn human from eight weeks of development to birth.

FRENCH KISSING (tongue kissing). While kissing, a person puts her or his tongue in the other person's mouth. French kissing includes using the tip of the tongue or the entire tongue.

FOREPLAY. Affectionate kissing, hugging and caressing/stimulating sexual organs between a couple prior to sexual intercourse.

FORESKIN. Hood-like piece of skin covering the tip of the uncircumcised penis.

FRATERNAL TWINS. Two separate ovum are fertilized and grow in the uterus. Fraternal twins may not have identical looks and they can be same sex twins or opposite sex twins.

GAY. Another term for male homosexuals; also used to describe both male and female homosexuals.

GENETIC. Pertaining to hereditary characteristics transferred from parents to children by way of chromosomes found in sperm and ova.

GENITALIA (genitals). Human external sex organs.

GENTIAL WARTS. STD. (See page 154.)

GESTATION. Period of carrying off spring in the uterus from conception to birth.

GLANS. Head of penis.

GONORRHEA. STD. (See page 155.)

HEPITITIS (Type B). STD. (See page 155.)

HERPES. A common STD (viral) which can cause harm to mother and baby. Herpes usually appears in the form of sores on the genitals.

HEMORRHOIDS. Irritating and sometimes painful swollen vein clusters outside or inside your anus (rectum). Minor hemorrhoids can be treated with non-prescription hemorrhoid creams, warm baths, exercise, proper diet, weight maintenance. Major hemorrhoids may require surgery. Child birth and strenuous exercise are frequent causes.

HETEROSEXUAL. Person who is sexually attracted to persons of the other sex—males attracted to females, females attracted to males.

HOMOSEXUAL. Person who is sexually attracted to members of her or his same sex.

HORMONE. A substance produced in one part of the body and transported by bodily fluids to another part of the body where it has a specific effect.

HYMEN. Thin piece of skin that may block or partially block the vaginal opening. Hymen structure varies greatly and some women are born without hymens.

HYSTERECTOMY. Surgery that removes a female's uterus and/or the ovaries and fallopian tubes for health reasons such as severe menstrual problems and pre-cancerous cell detection.

IDENTICAL TWINS. The fertilized ovum splits creating two separate same sex, identical-looking embryos. Twins are usually born within a few minutes of each other.

INCEST. Any sexual activity (including oral sex or intercourse) between family members other than husband-wife sexual relations. Incest is a crime. Incest most often occurs between parent and child or between siblings.

INFERTILITY (sterility). In women, the inability to become pregnant; in men the inability to produce sufficient sperm for conception.

LABIA (lips). The two flaps of skin on each side of the vaginal opening.

LESBIAN. A female who is sexually attracted to other females.

MAKING OUT (necking). Prolonged kissing sessions.

MASOCHISM. A degrading sexual exploitation in which a person receives pleasure from being abused or dominated by another person (masochist—the person suffering).

MASTURBATION (slang: jacking, jerking or beating off, playing with yourself, beating your meat). Self-stimulating one's clitoris or penis, usually to the point of orgasm.

MENARCHE. Medical term for a girl's first menstrual period.

MENSES. Blood and dead cells discharged from the uterus through the vagina each month during menstruation.

MENSTRUATION (slang: period, on the rag). Monthly shedding of unfertilized ovum and uterine lining of non-pregnant females.

MISCARRIAGE. See Abortion.

NOCTURNAL EMISSION (wet dream). Semen released from the penis while a male is asleep.

ORAL SEX (cunnilingus, fellatio) (slang: blow job, 69ing, giving head, eating at the y.). A form of sexual expression in which one person stimulates another person's sexual organs by using her or his mouth and tongue.

ORGASM (climax) (slang: cuming/coming). The moment of sexual stimulation when the nerve endings in the penis or clitoris register an eruption of pleasurable feeling.

OVARIES. Sex glands in the female where ova are stored.

OVARIAN CYST. An abnormal growth of cells on an ovary. Usually treated by high-estrogen contraceptives to shrink the growth or removed by surgery. Symptoms may include mild to severe abdominal pain and missed periods.

PMS. (Premenstrual Syndrome). A group of physical and emotional symptoms that precede a menstrual period, such as fluid retention, fatigue, irritability, depression and headache.

PENIS. Male sex organ that releases urine from the bladder and also deposits sperm in the female vagina during intercourse.

PHALLIC SYMBOL. Term used to refer to any object, shaped like an erect penis.

PLACENTA (afterbirth). Spongy mass of blood and tissue nurturing the embryo and fetus during development; expelled after birth of baby.

PORNOGRAPHY. Sexually-explicit written or visual material created for the purpose of sexual stimulation or sexual perversion.

PREGNANCY. In human females the condition of a fertilized ovum attached to the uterus. Carrying a developing fetus.

PROGESTERONE. A female hormone, also synthetically produced for contraceptive use in the Pill.

PROSTRATE GLAND. Male sex gland that produces semen.

PUBERTY. Growth stage (usually between ages ten to nineteen) in which a person's child body develops into their adult body including the maturing of their reproductive system.

PUBIC HAIR. Male and female genital hair.

PUBIC LICE. STD. (See page 155.)

RAPE. A sex crime punishable by law in which a person forces another person to have intercourse.

S & M. Abbreviation for sadism and masochism.

STDs (sexually transmitted diseases). Harmful diseases that are transmitted from one partner to another by sexual (vaginal, oral and anal) intercourse.

SADISM. Degrading sexual exploitation in which a person receives pleasure from sexually abusing or dominating another person (sadist —person inflicting the pain).

SADOMASOCHISM. Degrading sexual exploitation in which a person receives pleasure from inflicting sexual pain on oneself and others. (sadomasochist).

SCROTUM. Sac of skin that houses the male testicles.

SEMEN. Sticky white liquid containing sperm that is ejaculated from the penis during intercourse, masturbation, or wet dreams.

SEXUAL INTERCOURSE (copulating, coupling) (slang: making love, doing it, going all the way, screwing, fucking, humping, poking). Insertion of the erect male penis into the female's vagina.

SIAMESE TWINS. Twins whose bodies are physically joined together at birth—a rare occurrence.

SPERM. Male reproductive cell that fertilizes the female's ovum (female reproductive cell) for the creation of new human life.

SPERMICIDE. Sperm-killing chemical in contraceptive foams, cremes and jellies to kill sperm, thus preventing conception.

SPONTANEOUS ERECTION. Uncontrollable erection of the penis for no apparent reason.

STILLBIRTH. A baby that is born dead because of a malfunction in development or delivery. With good prenatal care, stillbirths rare.

SYPHILIS. STD. (See page 155.)

TESTOSTERONE. The male sex hormone.

TRANSVESTITE. A person who enjoys wearing the other sex's clothing.

TRICHOMONIASIS. STD. (See page 155.)

TOXIC SHOCK SYNDROME (TSS). A rare but serious, sometimes fatal disease caused by improper use of tampons and contraceptive sponges.

TUBAL LIGATION. Surgery in which a female's fallopian tubes are tied so ova and sperm can't unite. This is a permanent form of contraception.

UTERUS (womb). Muscular, pear-shaped, sex organ in the female that houses the fetus as it grows and develops.

VAGINA (slang: cunt, pussy, box, hole, snatch). Passageway of tough elastic muscle leading from the external genitalia to the uterus.

VAGINITIS. An itching or burning inflammation of the vagina and vulva which can be caused by a variety of symptoms including yeast infections, and STDs.

VASECTOMY. Permanent contraceptive method for men who do not want to father any/or more children; surgery where the vas deferens is cut to prevent sperm from mixing with the semen.

VENEREAL DISEASE. See STD.

VIRGIN. Man or woman who has not experienced sexual intercourse.

VULVA. External genital organs of female.

WET DREAM. See Nocturnal emission

WITHDRAWAL. The male pulling his penis out of the female's vagina before ejaculation—withdrawal is not a form of birth control. Pulling out is useless since sperm from pre-ejaculatory semen from the end of the penis is already in the vagina.

WOMB. See Uterus

Additional Reading

Bell, Ruth. *Changing Bodies, Changing Lives, A Book For Teens On Sex And Relationships*. New York: Random House, 1980, 1987.

Brothers, Joyce. *What Every Woman Ought To Know About Love & Marriage*. New York: Ballantine Books, 1984.

Cassell, Carol. *Straight from the Heart—How to talk to your teenagers about love and sex*. New York: Simon and Schuster, 1987.

Carlson, Dale. *Boys Have Feelings Too, Growing Up Male for Boys*. New York: Athenaeum, 1980.

Gordon, Sol and Judith. *Raising a Child Conservatively in a Sexually Permissive World*. New York: Simon and Schuster, 1983.

Johnson, Earwin "Magic". *What You Can Do to Avoid AIDS*. New York: Times Books, 1992.

Madaras, Lynda. *The What's Happening To My Body? Book For Girls*. New York: Newmarket Press, 1983, 1988.

Planned Parenthood. *How to Talk with Your Child about Sexuality —a Parent's Guide*. New York: Doubleday, 1986.

Rush, Florence. *The Best Kept Secret, Sexual Abuse of Children*. New York: McGraw-Hill Book Company, 1980.

Short, Ray E. *Sex, Love or Infatuation: How can I really know?* Minneapolis: Augsburg Publishing House, 1978.

Silverstein, Herma. *Teenage and Pregnant, What You Can Do.* Englewood Cliffs, NJ: Julian Messner a division of Silver Burdett Press, Inc., 1988.

Tribe, Lawrence H. *Abortion; the Clash of Absolutes.* New York: Norton, 1990.

Weisman, Michael and Betsy. *What We Told Our Kids About Sex.* New York: Harcourt Brace Jovanovich, 1987.

Index

228 **Index**

About the Author

Cynthia G. Akagi is the mother of two children, a daughter and a son. She is assistant director, Shawnee County Teen Pregnancy Prevention Program, Topeka, Kansas. Cynthia teaches parent-preteen sexuality classes and workshops, facilitates Teen Jams, serves as an educational liaison to area schools and writes a monthly sexuality column Talking With Teens.

Books by
GYLANTIC PUBLISHING

Teenage Addicts Can Recover: Treating The Addict, Not The Age

Shelly Marshall

Treatment providers & parents; 160 pages; $12.95; ISBN 1-880197-02-2, softcover
"Teenage treatment centers aren't working," says Ms. Marshall. The long term recovery rate for teenage addicts is less than 5%. Emphasizes the benefits of multi-generational treatment—improved recovery rates and cost savings for parents and society. Covers identifying the addict teen, choosing the best recovery program and post-treatment care, a necessary but slighted aspect of keeping teens living drug free in today's environment. Illustrations–Bibliography–Index

AMEND Philosophy And Curriculum For Treating Batterers

Michael Lindsey, Robert W. McBride and Constance M. Platt

For treatment providers; 124 pages; $16.95; ISBN 1-880197-04-9, softcover
Abusive Men Exploring New Directions (AMEND). Philosophy and treatment necessary to work with perpetrators. Covers male gender training and battering, values-laden versus values-free therapy, characteristics of batterers, character disorders, aggression, the battering relationship, containment. Talks about procedures—the intake of court-ordered clients, therapeutic contract, first contact, obsessional thinking, crisis intervention, and the group process. Charts & Illustrations–Index

AMEND Workbook For Ending Violent Behavior

Michael Lindsey, Robert W. McBride and Constance M. Platt

For clients; 100 pages; $11.95; ISBN 1-880197-05-7, softcover
This is a tool for men in treatment for domestic violence. It addresses the perpetrator directly. The information and exercises challenge his ideas, allow him to think about how he lives his life, encourages discussion in therapy, and helps him develop skills to improve his life. Index

Set: AMEND Philosophy And Curriculum For Treating Batterers
AMEND Workbook For Ending Violent Behavior

For treatment providers and educators; $28.90, ISBN 1-880197-06-5, softcover

The String on a Roast Won't Catch Fire in the Oven: An A-Z Encyclopedia Of Common Sense For The Newly Independent Young Adult

Candice Kohl

Young adults; 190 pages; $12.95; ISBN 1-880197-07-3, softcover
The String... provides young adults with a source of practical information they might have missed—the unexpected expenses of renting an apartment; organizing a simple budget; maintaining a checking account; food shopping and storing basics; housekeeping; quality and cost; and ends with a potpourri of helpful hints. Resources–Index

Moving With Children: A Parent's Guide To Moving With Children

Thomas Olkowski, Ph.D. and Lynn Parker, LCSW

Parents; 196 pages; $12.95; ISBN 1-880197-08-1, softcover
Moving... helps parents understand and deal with the many feelings and behaviors of children when families move. Practical and effective suggestions to help families deal with the various stages of moving—from planning and discussing the move with their children to saying goodbye, packing and unpacking, exploring the new community, meeting new friends, and settling into the new home. Helps parents create a spirit of emotional support and teamwork with their children. Resources, Bibiolgraphy, Illustrations, Index.

Helper: Real Stories of Welfare

Sonya Jason
Social workers and politicians; 158 pag

Helper shows what doesn't work and wha~~t needs to change~~
costly civilian bureaucracies, welfare and probation. *Helper* is a series of vignettes about people and situations as seen through the eyes of the author who as a social worker and probation officer spent years working with people and the bureaucracies that were suppose to help them. The stories depict the wonder and diversity of human beings and the looniness of bureaucracies determined to fit people into rigid slots and deal with them accordingly. Sometimes the people are amusing, sometimes dangerous.

Dear Larissa: Sexuality Education for Girls Ages 11-17

Cynthia G. Akagi
Girls ages 11-17; 242 pages, $12.95; ISBN 1-880197-10-3, softcover
A book for mothers (fathers) to give to their daughters. It is a mother's letters to her daughter about growing up—body changes, menstruation, boys, dating, love and sex—with space for personal comments. Many parents and their children are not comfortable discussing sexuality issues. *Dear Larissa* helps parents and daughters build communication in a caring manner. A book to be read and referred to by girls ages 11 through 17. Illustrations, Glossary, Bibliography, Index.

The Power of Touch: A Guide to Healing Sexual Abuse Through Poetry Therapy

Shelly Marshall and Kiley Kiebert   Publication date: Spring 1994
Young survivors of sexual abuse; 70 pages*, $ 7.95, ISBN 1-880197-11-1, softcover
The Power of Touch is a powerful self-help workbook of poetry therapy designed for victims of childhood sexual abuse. The book is organized in two parts—prose and poetry which is read first and a workbook which follows. The workbook is in three sections corresponding to body, mind/emotions and spirit. The theme is validation: This happened to me; this is how I think and feel about it; this is how I become whole again.

* Page count not firm at this printing

Prices valid in the United States only and subject to change without notice.

These bestsellers are available in your bookstore or order by calling, toll-free,
1-800-828-0113 to use your Visa/MasterCard.

Mail orders must include *complete payment* (check or Visa/MasterCard number with expiration date) unless you are a government agency, college, library or another official public organization, in which case please include a purchase order number.

Include $2.00 for shipping & handling with each order.
Colorado residents need to also include 3.8% sales tax.

To ensure your order is properly handled, include the name and quantity of each title, your complete name and shipping address and complete payment. Thank you.

Send orders to: GYLANTIC PUBLISHING CO.   (303) 797-6093
P. O. Box 2792   FAX 727-4279
Littleton, CO 80161-2792